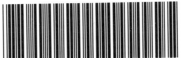

369 0246890

Colorectal Cancer in the Elderly

Kok-Yang Tan

Editor

Colorectal Cancer in the Elderly

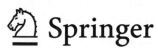 Springer

Editor

K.-Y. Tan, MBBS(Melb), MMed(Surg),
FRCS, FAMS
Department of General Surgery
Geriatric Surgery Service
Khoo Teck Puat Hospital
Alexandra Health
Singapore

ISBN 978-3-642-29882-0   ISBN 978-3-642-29883-7   (eBook)
DOI 10.1007/978-3-642-29883-7
Springer Heidelberg New York Dordrecht London

Library of Congress Control Number: 2012947996

Printed on acid-free paper

Springer is part of Springer Science+Business Media (www.springer.com)

Special Dedication

This book is dedicated to the patients that continue to inspire us to do better.

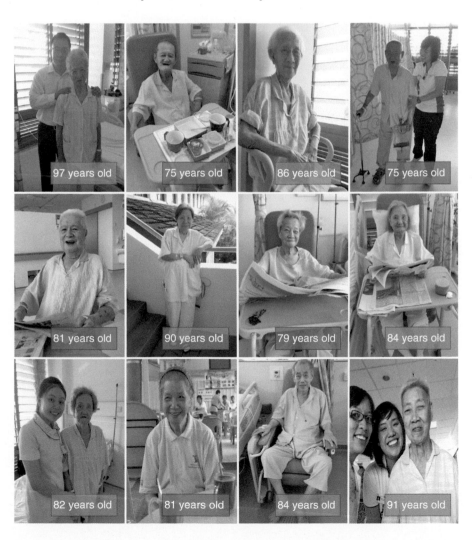

Contents

The Normal Physiology of Aging

1

Kenneth Mak

Take Home Pearls

- Aging causes biological changes in the organ systems which reduce functional capacity and reserve.
- The elderly patient may present with disease in atypical ways.
- Adjustments in the treatment plan need to be done to take effects of aging into account.

1.1   Introduction

Aging refers to the complex biological changes that progressively occur over time, affecting most organ systems in the human body. These anatomic and physiologic changes often lead to a gradual decline in functional capacity with increasing age. The physiologic reserve of the older patient is progressively depleted, leading to an increase in susceptibility to disease as well as an increasing vulnerability to external insults.

The decrease in physiologic reserve is not always immediately evident in the healthy elderly patient. However, in times of illness, the diminished functional reserve leads to the older patient not being able to mount an adequate compensatory response to an insult, whether from environmental hazards, disease or injury. They also have a diminished ability to tolerate major surgery. When complications arise, these complications often have a more severe impact on the elderly patient compared to the younger patient and lead to a more adverse outcome.

K. Mak
Department of General Surgery, Khoo Teck Puat Hospital,
Singapore, Singapore
e-mail: mak.kenneth.sw@alexandrahealth.com.sg

K.-Y. Tan (ed.), *Colorectal Cancer in the Elderly*,
DOI 10.1007/978-3-642-29883-7_1, © Springer-Verlag Berlin Heidelberg 2013

1

The physiologic changes in the older patient may also lead to the patient exhibiting atypical clinical features, or minimal clinical features, when presenting with illness (Boss and Seegmiller 1981). This can lead to a delayed diagnosis or a failure to appreciate the severity of the clinical disease. This chapter gives an overview of some of the physiological changes occurring in the various body systems of the elderly system and its clinical implications.

1.2   Aging and the Cardiovascular System

The aging heart undergoes various structural changes. This includes a decrease in the overall number of cardiac muscle cells, an increased deposition of collagen and formation of cross-linkages between the cardiac muscle fibres. Although systolic function and resting cardiac output is usually well preserved in the healthy aging heart, these structural changes in the cardiac muscle contribute to an impairment in diastolic relaxation and the filling of the heart during diastole. There is an increased risk of diastolic dysfunction and diastolic heart failure.

The aging cardiac muscle also has a reduced inotropic response to beta-adrenergic stimulation. As such, the elderly patient has blunted heart rate and myocardial contractility responses to catecholamines, whether of exogenous or endogenous origin. The aging heart is unable to mount a compensatory tachycardia as efficiently as in the younger patient, when by exercise or in haemodynamic shock states. This leads to a significant decrease in peak cardiac output by 20–30% in the elderly patient. The cardiac muscle cells also have a lowered inotropic response to digoxin, making such drugs less effective when used in the elderly patient.

Age-related changes are also present in the conduction system in the heart. There is an increased risk of sinus node dysfunction, with an associated increase in the duration of the refractory interval as well as a slowing of the conduction pathways within the heart. These changes lead to an increase propensity for dysrhythmias in the elderly. These dysrhythmias may arise spontaneously or under stressed conditions, e.g. in sepsis.

Changes also occur within the blood vessels of the healthy elderly patient. An increased arterial stiffness is often observed in the elderly patient. This causes the arteries to have reduced distensibility, which leads to an increase in the pulse wave velocity throughout the vascular system and contributes to a rise in the systemic vascular resistance. As the afterload of the heart increases, secondary changes may arise in the cardiac myocardium, causing left ventricular hypertrophy. The changes in the blood vessels can arise independent of any associated hypertension or atherosclerotic disease. The same aging blood vessels have altered endothelial function, and the vasoactive responses to both alpha- and beta- adrenergic stimulation are attenuated.

The physiologic changes affecting the aging heart and vascular system are often overshadowed by the higher prevalence of atherosclerotic disease, hypertension, valvular heart disease and coronary artery disease in the elderly population. The combined influence of the physiologic changes arising in the aging heart, coupled with increased incidence of comorbid cardiac disease, leads to the aging patient having a greater perioperative cardiac risk.

1.3   Aging and the Respiratory System

Worsening respiratory function is often seen in the elderly patient, and this is the result of changes in both the lung and chest wall.

The chest wall of the elderly patient is stiffer, due to calcification of the ribs and the vertebral joints. The thoracic cage thus expands less during inspiration. Age-related kyphosis may arise, due to osteoporosis and an increased vulnerability to vertebral compression fractures. This further limits chest wall expansion and places the diaphragm in a mechanically disadvantageous position in relation to the chest wall, leading to less effective contractions. Lung compliance is further compromised by a decrease in pulmonary surfactant production in the elderly patient (Brandsletter and Kazemi 1983). The overall volume-pressure curve of the lungs and thorax is flattened and an associated increase in work of breathing results.

Respiratory muscle strength progressively deteriorates with increasing age. This is due to a combination of factors, including a decrease in respiratory muscle mass, motor neuronal loss within the muscles, impairment in calcium pump activity within the sarcoplasmic reticulum and decline in mitochondrial respiratory chain function. This problem may be exacerbated by poor feeding and malnutrition in the elderly, and contributes to rapid deconditioning. The elderly patient in intensive care is also at increased risk for ventilator dependence with difficulty experienced in weaning of the ventilator.

Within the respiratory bronchioles and alveolar ducts, loss of collagen and elastin with increasing age leads to a progressive enlargement of these airways (Close and Woodson 1989). The widening of the airways is associated with a corresponding decrease in volume of air within the alveoli. The functional alveolar surface area available for gaseous exchange can decrease by as much as 15%, by the age of 70 years. Closing volume is the lung volume at which the airways begin to close during expiration and this increases with age. As a result of this change in closing volume and expansion in the volume of air in the airways, an increase in physiologic dead space results and contributes to ventilation – perfusion mismatch within the lungs.

A gradual increase in residual volume and an associated decrease in vital capacity occur as a person ages. The functional residual capacity (FRC) also increases progressively with age (Janssens et al. 1999). A decrease in the volume of the pulmonary capillary bed with aging is often associated with an increase in pulmonary arterial pressures and pulmonary vascular resistance.

Control of breathing is also adversely affected in the elderly. The central and peripheral chemoreceptor response to hypercapnia is blunted. Thus, elderly patients are more susceptible to apnoeic and hypoxaemic episodes during their sleep.

Depression of the protective upper airway reflexes occurs with advancing age. A greater amount of stimulation is required to trigger the protective reflexes. Neurologic disorders can exacerbate this impairment in the airway protective reflexes and increase the risk of pulmonary aspiration (Sharma and Goodwin 2006).

1.4   Aging and the Renal System

Both structural damage and functional decline occur in the aging kidneys. The progressive decline in renal function may not lead to significant clinical impact in a healthy elderly patient due to the initial high amount of redundancy and functional reserve in the kidneys. However, when exposed to disease and medical therapies, the diminished physiologic reserve may lead to acute deterioration in renal function in stressed states.

A steady decrease in renal mass of about 20% occurs in healthy individuals between the ages of 30 and 80 years. Renal blood flow is initially preserved up to the fourth decade of life but subsequently decreases steadily at a rate of approximately 10% per decade of life (Beck 1998). This decline is associated by a 50% reduction in glomerular filtration rate, by the age of 90 years. Tubular function similarly decreases with progressive age. There is impaired handling of sodium, potassium and acid load excretion, as well as in fluid handling and renal drug excretion (McLean and Le Couteur 2004).

Because of these age-related changes in renal physiology, the elderly patient is more susceptible to perioperative fluid and electrolyte imbalances. Hyponatraemia is more common in the elderly, may arise as a result of an intrinsic impaired ability of the aging kidney to excrete free water and exacerbated by a combination of influences, including age-related higher levels of ADH, lower levels of renin and aldosterone, inadequate dietary intake of sodium, diuretic-induced renal dysfunction and increased sodium losses if diarrhoea or vomiting were to be present (Lubran 1995).

Paying close attention to the intra-operative volume status, avoiding haemodynamic lability and the use of nephrotoxic drugs is critical to minimising post-operative renal deterioration in the older patient.

1.5   Aging and the Hepatobiliary System

Compared to other organs in the body, the aging liver is better able to preserve its function despite structure changes. The capacity of the liver to regenerate is fairly well maintained in the elderly patient but may occur at a slower pace.

The aging liver undergoes brown atrophy, characterised histologically by an accumulation of lipofuscin granules in the hepatocytes. A reduction in size of the liver occurs, with increase in the amount of fibrous tissue deposition within the liver. There is also a corresponding decrease in hepatic and splanchnic blood flow. The decline in hepatocyte mass and hepatic perfusion, together with age-related changes in the hepatic sinusoidal endothelium, influences hepatic drug metabolism and clearance (Anantharaju et al. 2002). Drugs with high liver extraction ratios (e.g. amiodarone, amitriptylline, diltiazem, fentanyl, labetalol, midazolam, propofol, nifedipine and verapamil) have impaired hepatic clearance in the elderly patient. Dynamic measurements of liver function, e.g. ICG clearance tests, demonstrate the gradual decline in liver function with aging better than conventional liver biochemistry tests, as the conventional "liver function test" often fails to demonstrate any significant age-specific change.

Aging of the liver is also associated with mitochondrial dysfunction and decreased intra-hepatic energy content. This renders the aging liver less tolerant of ischaemic insults. The risk of liver dysfunction and failure is thus higher in the critically ill elderly surgical patient. Ischaemic pre-conditioning and similar liver-protective strategies have less efficacy in the elderly.

Biliary duct ectasia in the biliary duct often arises with aging. The calibre of the extra-hepatic biliary ducts thus is generally bigger in the elderly patient. Lithogenicity of bile salts tends to increase with aging, contributing to an increased tendency for gallstone development.

1.6   Aging and the Gut

Anorexia is often observed in the elderly patient and is due to a variety of influences, including impaired smell and taste, altered gastric fundal compliance, altered secretion of gastrointestinal hormones, changes in the autonomic nervous system feedback to the central nervous system, as well as alterations in the levels of leptin and steroid hormones (Morley 2007).

The older patient may have a prolonged oropharyngeal phase in swallowing and a delay in the opening of the upper oesophageal sphincter. A greater amount of fluid is necessary to induce the pharyngeal swallows in the older patient and stimulate the pharyngo-gluttal closure reflex. These abnormalities in the swallowing reflex are particularly significant, if a concomitant lack of protective reflexes arises, e.g. due to a bulbar palsy. An increased risk of pulmonary aspiration then results.

Age-related changes in oesophageal function (otherwise known as presbyesophagus) may also arise, due primarily to impairment of oesophageal motility. An overall decrease in peristalsis and a delay in transit time occur in the elderly patient. There is also an increased incidence of non-peristaltic contractions in the lower oesophagus and diminished relaxation of the lower oesophageal sphincter on swallowing, which can lead to dysphagia.

The elderly patient has a higher incidence of atrophic gastritis, and this may be due to changes in gastric acid production.

Changes in the commensal intestinal microflora may occur in the older patient. There is a decrease in the total number of bifidobacteria. Fungi and enterobacteria tend to proliferate more. These changes in the intestinal microflora contribute to an increase propensity for the critically ill elderly patient to develop Clostridium difficile-related pseudomembranous colitis and diarrhoea.

A gradual decrease in intestinal motility is often observed in the elderly patient. This leads to a prolonged stool transit time, greater stool dehydration and chronic constipation. On the other hand, the elderly patient may also experience loss of tone in the external rectal sphincter and, this can lead to faecal incontinence.

A gradual decline in pancreatic exocrine output may arise with aging. These changes may not lead to an appreciable impairment in fat or protein digestion and absorption in the healthy elderly patient but may be significant in contributing to malnutrition in sickness.

1.7 Aging and the Endocrine System

The aging process affects nearly every endocrine gland in the body. For example, there is impaired secretion of hypothalamic hormones and an impaired pituitary response to the same hormones. Decline in hypothalamic function, together with a lowered basal metabolic rate and changes in the thermoregulatory threshold for peripheral vasoconstriction and shivering, leads to the body being less able to generate and conserve heat. The elderly patient is now more vulnerable to hypothermia in a cold environment. Febrile responses are also blunted and can pose a diagnostic challenge as the elderly patient may not mount a fever when presenting with sepsis.

The pituitary gland is smaller and more fibrous in the elderly patient. An age-related decrease in growth hormone production may lead to decrease lean muscle mass (sarcopaenia), decreased heart function and contribute to osteoporosis.

A blunted response by the thyroid gland to thyroid stimulating hormone (TSH) can result in a decrease in the production of thyroid hormone. Clinical hypothyroidism, which occurs in 10% if females and 2% of males above the age of 60 years, can lead to a decrease in basal metabolic rate and is an important cause of chronic constipation in the elderly (Rehman et al. 2005).

Aging is also associated with a progressive decline in insulin secretion as well as increasing insulin resistance. This predisposes the elderly individual to impaired glucose tolerance and diabetes. Sarcopaenia as well as an increase in both body and visceral fat is some of the changes in body composition observed in elderly patients. This arises due to a combination of factors, including decreased physical activity, declining endocrine function and increased insulin resistance.

Endocrine failure in the aging ovaries leads to menopause. In menopause, the ovaries stop responding to follicle stimulating hormone (FSH) and luteinizing hormone from the anterior pituitary gland. Ovarian production of oestrogen and progesterone decreases and eventually ceases. This leads to the clinical aspects of menopause, namely, the absence of further menses.

Androgen deficiency, or late onset hypogonadism, affects as much as 30% of men in their 60s and 50% of all men above the age of 80 years. This contributes to changes in body composition, osteoporosis, cognitive decline and erectile dysfunction (Shelton and Rajfer 2012).

1.8 Aging and the Skin

Atrophic changes occur in the skin with advancing age. The epidermis atrophies and the turnover rate of cells in the stratum corneum decrease. Decreases in epidermal cell growth and division lead to slower skin re-epithelisation as well as delayed wound healing. Aging skin is less prone to hypertrophied scar and keloid formation. The thinner skin is more vulnerable to injury and ischaemia. The elderly patient is particularly at risk of decubitus ulcers when kept immobile for prolonged period.

The dermal collagen is stiffer and less pliable in the elderly patient. The elastin is also more cross-linked and has a higher amount of calcification. These changes lead to a loss of skin tone and elasticity, contributing to skin wrinkling and sagging. The subcutaneous blood vessels are more fragile and tend to be injured more easily with minor trauma or pressure. Thus, bruising is more common in the elderly.

Aging skin tends to be more dry, due to reduced sweat production and oil secretion. Superficial skin infections are more frequent in the elderly, in part due to the change in the local milieu within the skin, encouraging more pathogenic bacteria to colonise the skin.

1.9   Aging and the Musculoskeletal System

A gradual decline in lean body mass, or sarcopaenia, occurs commonly with aging. This is primarily due to a loss and atrophy of muscle cells. The elderly patient is easily deconditioned if he is subject to prolonged immobilisation. Changes in the innervation of muscles may contribute to decreased muscular function. An increase in body fat is also observed in the older patient.

Osteoporosis is commonly seen in the elderly patient. This is characterised by a net loss in bone rather than a decrease in the ratio of mineral to matrix (as in osteomalacia). Osteoporosis leads to decreased strength and an increased susceptibility to fractures, with a lower applied force (Simon 2005). The osteoporotic fractures tend to have a characteristic age-dependent pattern of incidence – wrist fractures tend to occur in the late 50s and early 60s, vertebral fractures in the 60s and 70s, and hip fractures in the 70s and 80s.

1.10   Aging and the Immune System

A general decline in immune competence may be seen in the elderly patient. This is characterised by an increase in susceptibility to infections as well as an increase in autoantibodies and monoclonal immunoglobulins. Changes in T-cell populations may be observed, with an associated decline in T-cell responsiveness to a variety of antigens. A resulting anergy can be demonstrated through delayed hypersensitivity skin tests.

1.11   A Loss of Functional Reserve Leads to Frailty

A decrease in physiological reserve results from the age-related changes in the different organ systems of the body. While this decrease in functional reserve often does not lead to a deterioration in the quality of life of a healthy elderly patient, the older patient is now placed metaphorically on the edge of a precipice. Disease and complications arising from medical treatment or surgery may present an insult against which the elderly patient is now unable to cope, due to his diminished reserve. As a result, he now falls off the precipice and may face a catastrophic adverse outcome.

It is important for clinicians looking after the elderly to be aware of the age-related changes that take place within their patients and to optimise clinical outcomes through avoiding insults that compromise the physiologic reserve of the elderly patient. A heightened awareness of the different manifestations of disease in the elderly and early diagnosis of surgical complications is critical to success.

References

Anantharaju A, Fellr A, Chedid A (2002) Aging liver. Gerontology 48(6):343–353
Beck LH (1998) Changes in renal function with aging. Clin Geriatr Med 14(2):199–209
Boss GR, Seegmiller JE (1981) Age-related physiological changes and their clinical significance. West J Med 135(6):434–440
Brandsletter RD, Kazemi H (1983) Aging and the respiratory system. Med Clin North Am 67(2):419–431
Close LG, Woodson GE (1989) Common upper airway disorders in the elderly and their management. Geriatrics 44(1):67–68, 71–62
Janssens JP, Pache JC, Nicod LP (1999) Physiologic changes in respiratory function associated with aging. Eur Respir J 13(1):197–205
Lubran MM (1995) Renal function in the elderly. Ann Clin Lab Sci 25(2):122–133
McLean AJ, Le Couteur DG (2004) Aging biology and geriatric clinical pharmacology. Pharmacol Rev 56(2):163–184
Morley JE (2007) The aging gut: physiology. Clin Geriatr Med 23(4):757–767
Rehman SU, Cope DW, Senseney AD, Brzezinski W (2005) Thyroid disorders in elderly patients. South Med J 98(5):543–549
Sharma G, Goodwin J (2006) Effect of aging on respiratory system physiology and immunology. Clin Interv Aging 1(3):253–260
Shelton JB, Rajfer J (2012) Androgen deficiency in aging and metabolically challenged men. Urol Clin North Am 39(1):63–75
Simon LS (2005) Osteoporosis. Clin Geriatr Med 21(3):603–629

Screening, Diagnosis, and Investigations for Colorectal Cancer in the Elderly

2

Shingo Tsujinaka and Yutaka J. Kawamura

Take Home Pearls

- Screening strategies in the elderly should be tailored to comorbid conditions and life expectancy.
- Colonoscopy in the elderly carries certain risks, regional safety data, and completion rates need to be taken into account when developing a screening strategy for a given population.
- The role of computed tomographic colonography remains uncertain.

2.1 Introduction

The incidence of colorectal cancer (CRC) increases with age. In the United States, a new diagnosis of CRC occurs in 24% in patients aged 64–74 years, 27% in those aged 75–84 years, and 12% in those aged 85 years or older (Day et al. 2011b). The US Preventive Services Task Force (USPSTF) recommended screening for CRC using fecal occult blood tests, sigmoidoscopy, or colonoscopy, beginning at the age of 50 years and continuing until age 75 years. The USPSTF recommends against routine screening for colorectal cancer in adults aged 76–85 years with individual consideration and recommends against any screening for those 85 years or older (2008). These distinctive recommendations may be attributable to unique characteristics of elderly

S. Tsujinaka (✉) • Y.J. Kawamura
Department of Surgery,
Jichi Medical University, Saitama Medical Center,
1-847, Amanumacho, Omiya, Saitama-shi,
Saitama 330-8503, Japan
e-mail: tsujinakas@omiya.jichi.ac.jp; kawamura@omiya.jichi.ac.jp

K.-Y. Tan (ed.), *Colorectal Cancer in the Elderly*,
DOI 10.1007/978-3-642-29883-7_2, © Springer-Verlag Berlin Heidelberg 2013

patients with more comorbid medical conditions, potential cognitive impairment resulting in informed consent difficulty, potential higher incidence of logistical problems (i.e., transportation), and shorter life expectancy compared with younger individuals (Lin et al. 2006). Some clinicians may have concerns in screening or diagnostic colonoscopy with regard to the possibility of inadequate bowel preparation, lower completion rate, and increased risk of adverse events (Lin et al. 2006).

This chapter highlights the efficacy and effectiveness, and the complex issues relative to CRC screening and subsequent investigative procedures.

2.2   Fecal Occult Blood Testing (FOBT)

2.2.1   Overview

FOBT is currently the most widely prescribed screening modality. Patients with positive FOBT results should undergo a follow-up complete colonoscopy, and previous trials have demonstrated that 15–33% reduction in colorectal cancer mortality can be achieved when positive FOBT results were followed by colonoscopy (Mandel et al. 1993; Hardcastle et al. 1996; Kronborg et al. 1996). Recommended tests for CRC screening in average-risk individuals beginning at age 50 years by guideline organizations include colonoscopy every 10 years as the most preferred modality, followed by annual fecal occult blood tests (FOBT), flexible sigmoidoscopy every 5 years, or annual FOBT plus flexible sigmoidoscopy every 5 years as alternatives (Davila et al. 2006).

FOBT can be typically performed with use of a guaiac-based test (G-FOBT) targeting peroxidase-like activity of hem or hemoglobin in feces, or immunochemical-based test (I-FOBT) using hemoglobin-specific antibodies (Davila et al. 2006). G-FOBT is highly sensitive but frequently affected by peroxidase-containing foods and dietary heme from red meat; 3-day food restrictions are necessary to avoid false-positive results. I-FOBT is more specific but less sensitive compared with G-FOBT; therefore, a combination of I-FOBT and G-FOBT should also be advocated to improve diagnostic accuracy (Allison et al. 1996; Greenberg et al. 2000).

2.2.2   FOBT Screening in the Elderly

Although FOBT screening is deemed to be effective in early detection, it may not benefit patients with short life expectancies since its benefit does not appear immediately (Walter and Covinsky 2001). This is reflected by the results from previous trials on FOBT aimed for reduction in mortality from CRC; the cancer-specific survival curves between the screened and unscreened patients did not differ significantly until at least 5 years after the initial screening (Mandel et al. 1993; Hardcastle et al. 1996; Kronborg et al. 1996). Cancers destined to result in death within 5 years of diagnosis may be too aggressive for patients to benefit from early detection and treatment, suggesting the elderly patients with estimated life expectancy of less than 5 years would not derive survival benefit from cancer screening (Walter and Covinsky 2001). The benefit of positive FOBT results from asymptomatic tumors must be weighed against immediate burdens of downstream procedures (i.e., colonoscopy) and treatments (i.e., endoscopic resection or surgical bowel resection) (Kistler et al. 2011).

2.3   Colonoscopy for Colorectal Cancer Screening in the Elderly

2.3.1   Overview

Colonoscopy is the preferred and the most common modality for CRC screening (Davila et al. 2006; Wexner et al. 2006). In order to achieve adequate inspection of the colonic mucosa, cathartic bowel preparation is necessary. When bowel preparation is given, it should be tolerable, safe, and effective, regardless of the age of the candidate.

2.3.2   Method of Bowel Preparation

A standard method of bowel cleansing is an ingestion of polyethylene glycol (PEG). Since PEG is nondigestible, nonabsorbable, and iso-osmolar with plasma, it only purges colonic luminal contents without affecting the physiologic conditions including body weights, blood pressures, and electrolytes (Day et al. 2011b; Juluri et al. 2011). The drawback of PEG is requirement of large volume of its solution (standard, 4 l; low volume, 2 l) and poor palatability. The former issue raises a particular concern to the elderly patients because inability to consume the prescribed treatment may affect the preparation quality (Thomson et al. 1996), although the estimated shortfall is considered to be relatively small with the reported mean volume consumption ranges from 91% to 93% (Belsey et al. 2007). The split dosing of PEG solution has been shown to be as effective as the whole dose protocol (El Sayed et al. 2003; Belsey et al. 2007; Cohen 2010); therefore, it may improve noncompliance rate in the elderly patients.

The common complaints in the elderly patients associated with PEG include dizziness, fecal incontinence, abdominal pain, and nausea (Day et al. 2011b). Also, there are case reports of adverse events such as pulmonary aspiration, pancreatitis, ischemic colitis, and dysnatremia in patients with impaired thirst sensation, suggesting the importance of adequate hydration during bowel preparation in these individuals (Day et al. 2011b).

The alternative method is the use of sodium phosphate (NaP). NaP consists of a low-volume laxative that osmotically draws plasma water into the bowel lumen to promote bowel cleansing (Wexner et al. 2006). NaP may be contraindicated for elderly patients because it can result in potentially fatal fluid shift and electrolyte disturbances (Curran and Plosker 2004; Lichtenstein et al. 2007). Also, patients taking angiotensin-converting enzyme inhibitors, angiotensin receptor blockers, diuretics, and nonsteroidal anti-inflammatory agents may have more adverse effects to bowel preparation for colonoscopy (Lichtenstein et al. 2007). In elderly patients, NaP appeared to be more

tolerated than PEG but had significantly more complications with electrolyte disturbances, with comparable quality of preparation (Thomson et al. 1996; Seinela et al.
2003). Furthermore, the recent prospective, randomized trial revealed that bowel
cleansing for colonoscopy using NaP induced tenfold likelihood of mucosal
inflammation than that of PEG (Lawrance et al. 2011). This finding may give further
caution to the selection of cathartic agents for colonoscopy in the elderly.

2.3.3 Complications During Colonoscopy

Colonoscopy-specific complications may potentially be fatal to the elderly patients
who are generally vulnerable to invasive procedure, and there has been controversy
over whether increased age is an independent risk factor (Day et al. 2011b). A recent
systematic review with meta-analysis (Day et al. 2011a) demonstrated that pooled
incidence of adverse events per 1,000 colonoscopies in patients 65 years of age and
older was as follows: 26.0 [95% CI, 25.0–27.0] for cumulative gastrointestinal (GI)
adverse events, 1.0 [95% CI, 0.9–1.5] for perforation, 6.3 [95% CI, 5.7–7.0] for
GI bleeding, 19.1 [95% CI, 18.0–20.3] for cardiovascular (CV)/pulmonary complications, and 1.0 [95% CI, 0.7–2.2] for mortality rate. Furthermore, among octogenarians, adverse events per 1,000 colonoscopies were as follows: 34.9 [95% CI, 31.9–38.0]
for cumulative GI adverse events, 1.5 [95% CI, 1.1–1.9] for perforation, 2.4 [95% CI,
1.1–4.6] for GI bleeding, 28.9 [95% CI, 26.2–31.8] for CV/pulmonary complications, and 0.5 [95% CI, 0.06–1.9] for mortality rate. These data indicate that patients
80 years of age and older have greater risk of cumulative GI adverse events and perforation compared with patients younger than 80 years of age. The incidence of
GI bleeding and CV/pulmonary complications tended to be higher in octogenarians
without statistical significance.

Although colonoscopy is generally considered a safe procedure, these results
should be integrated to discussions when considering colonoscopy, including informed
consent process, clinical decision making, and refining population-based screening
policies in the elderly (Day et al. 2011a).

2.3.4 Completion Rate of Colonoscopy

Completion rate in performing total colonoscopy is reportedly very high over 90%
(Day et al. 2011b); however, it appears to be lower in octogenarians with a mean of
84.7% ± 11.7% (Day et al. 2011a). Some studies included increased age as the factors predictive of failed colonoscopy or technical difficulty with prolonged cecal
intubation (Lukens et al. 2002; Schmilovitz-Weiss et al. 2007; Lee et al. 2008), while
some did not show that age directly associate with adjusted completion rate (Nelson
et al. 2002; Arora and Singh 2004; Karajeh et al. 2006) and the procedural failure
was rather affected by the higher prevalence of bowel stricture because of diverticular disease and/or malignancy (Karajeh et al. 2006) or poorer bowel preparation
(Nelson et al. 2002) in the elderly.

2.3.5 Japanese Perspectives on Colonoscopy

There have been a number of studies conducted by Japanese colonoscopists in an effort to improve cecal intubation rate, cecal intubation time, total examination time, and disease detection rate and to reduce complication rate and patient discomfort (Kondo et al. 2007; Tsutsumi et al. 2007; Horiuchi et al. 2008; Harada et al. 2009; Takeuchi et al. 2010). In one randomized controlled trial, the efficacy of the transparent hood attached to the colonoscope was assessed (Kondo et al. 2007). The overall cecal intubation rate was 96.4%, 94.3%, and 95.3% in the transparent hood, short hood, and no-hood groups, respectively ($p = 0.58$). Only a history of abdominal surgery had a significantly negative impact on successful cecal intubation in the multivariate analysis. Increased age (70 years of age or older) was not independently associated with completion of cecal intubation. However, the average cecal intubation time in patients aged 70 years or older was 13.5, 16.0, and 20.0 min in the transparent hood, short hood, and no-hood groups, respectively ($p = 0.04$). The use of the transparent hood was attributed to a 17% reduction in cecal intubation time ($p = 0.003$). This trial also showed that the use of the transparent hood was effective for trainee endoscopists in shortening cecal intubation time in difficult case such as elderly (70 years of age or older) and female patients. In another similar randomized trial (Harada et al. 2009), the mean cecal intubation time was significantly shorter in the hood group (10.2 min) than in the no-hood group (13.4 min). The proportion of examinees who answered comfortable was 35.9% in the hood group and 27.6% in the no-hood group ($p = 0.04$), and those who answered intolerable was 18.0% in the hood group and 25.4% in the no-hood group ($p = 0.037$). However, the cecal intubation rate did not differ between the hood group (96.5%) and the no-hood group (95.0%). Additionally, in a large retrospective study, the completion rate was 96.8% in patients less than 80 years of age compared with 92.7% in those aged 80 years or older (Tsutsumi et al. 2007). Furthermore, two studies showed very low complication rate in very old patients, 0.9% (bleeding after polypectomy) in octogenarians (Tsutsumi et al. 2007) and 1.7% (oxygen administration due to deep sedation) in nonagenarians (Horiuchi et al. 2008). The authors believe that these encouraging evidences have optimal roles in improved screening colonoscopy for the elderly population.

2.4 Current Issues in Colorectal Cancer Screening in the Elderly: The Net Benefit or the Net Burden?

Emerging literatures regarding benefits and burdens from CRC screening in the United States have impacted on the significance of existing screening strategy. In the setting where fewer than 60% of patients receive a colonoscopy within 1 year after positive FOBT result, elderly adults tend to have low rate of follow-up colonoscopy compared to younger patients (Kistler et al. 2011). A longitudinal study determining the frequency of downstream outcomes during 7 years of follow-up was conducted targeting 212 patients 70 years or older with a positive FOBT result at four Veteran Affairs facilities (Kistler et al. 2011). Fifty-six percent of patients received follow-up colonoscopy, detecting 34 significant adenomas and 6 cancers. In contrast, 46% of those without colonoscopy died of other causes (43 of 94), while three died of CRC within 5 years after FOBT. This study also showed that 87% of patients with the worst life expectancy experienced a net burden from screening (26 of 30) as did 70% with average life expectancy (92 of 131) and 65% with the best life expectancy (35 of 51). Thus, it is reasonably assumed that patients with the best life expectancy would benefit from screening more than those with the worst (Kistler et al. 2011), and this has been verified by the multi-modeling analyses (Ko and Sonnenberg 2005; Lin et al. 2006). One study compared the risk and benefits of screening in patients aged 70–94 years with differing health status using three screening strategies including annual fecal occult blood tests, flexible sigmoidoscopy every 5 years, or colonoscopy every 10 years (Ko and Sonnenberg 2005). One cancer-related death would be prevented by screening 42 healthy men aged 70–74 years with colonoscopy, 178 healthy women aged 70–74 years with fecal occult blood tests, 431 women aged 75–79 years in poor health with colonoscopy, or 945 men aged 80–84 years in average health with fecal occult blood tests. These results indicate that the potential benefits and risks of screening vary in elderly patients of different life expectancies (Ko and Sonnenberg 2005). The other showed that the prevalence of colonic neoplasia increased with age; however, screening colonoscopy in elderly patients (patients 80 years of age and older) resulted in only 15% of the expected gain in life expectancy in younger patients (patients 50–54 years of age), even when adjusted for life expectancy (Lin et al. 2006).

Nevertheless, it is importantly advised that the aforementioned estimated life expectancy is based on the populations in the United States; therefore, difference in life years saved by screening may vary in different geographic locations such as Europe, Asia, and other nations (Day et al. 2011b).

Overuse of screening colonoscopy is another issue that may associate with procedural adverse effects and increased expenditures using limited resources (Goodwin et al. 2011). Among 24,071 Medicare patients with a negative initial screening colonoscopy, 46% underwent a repeated colonoscopy in fewer than 7 years, including 46% of patients aged 75–79 years and 33% of those aged 89 years or older. These results clearly did not meet the available universal guidelines (Davila et al. 2006). Moreover, in 43% of patients who had a repeated colonoscopy, there was no clear indication for repeated examination. In their multivariate analyses, interestingly, male sex, more comorbidities, and colonoscopy by a high-volume colonoscopist or in an office setting were associated with higher rates of the early repeated examination without clear indication (Goodwin et al. 2011). To explain this, the authors presumed that patients with multiple comorbidities see more medical providers and thus increasing their opportunities of being recommended for another screening colonoscopy, though it is generally perceived that the presence of comorbid medical conditions reduces the benefit of CRC screening (Day et al. 2011b).

2.5   Potential Role of Computed Tomographic Colonography (CTC)

Although preimaging bowel preparation using cathartic agents is still necessary, computed tomographic colonography (CTC) is currently available as minimally invasive procedure for detection of colonic neoplasia (Heresbach et al. 2011).

A recent meta-analysis assessing the diagnostic value of CTC for screening demonstrated that estimated per patient sensitivity of CTC for greater than or equal to 6-mm polyps and adenomas were 68.1% and 78.6%, with the corresponding specificity of 94.6% or 91.4%, whereas the estimated per patient sensitivity for greater than or equal to 10-mm polyps and adenomas were 83.3% and 87.9%, with the corresponding specificity of 98.7% and 97.6% (de Haan et al. 2011). This meta-analysis concluded that CTC has a high sensitivity for adenomas greater than or equal to 10 mm and has lower sensitivity for adenomas greater than or equal to 6 mm, as compared to colonoscopy (de Haan et al. 2011).

Macari et al. (2011) undertook a retrospective cohort study comparing the frequency of recommendations for additional imaging (RAIs) for extracolonic findings, polyp prevalence among seniors (65 years of age and older) and non-seniors (younger than 65 years of age). The polyp prevalence was similar (14.2% for seniors vs. 13.2% for non-seniors), and the presence of extracolonic findings was significantly more frequent in seniors than in non-seniors (74.0% vs. 55.4%) but without statistical significance in RAIs (6.0% in seniors vs. 4.4% in non-seniors).

Since the tagging technique of residual colonic material allows discriminate high-density stool and fluid from the colonic wall, CT colonography may not require rigorous bowel cleansing compared with colonoscopy (Keedy et al. 2011). As a result, lesser volume of cathartic agents can improve patient adherence and tolerability, and the optimal solutions of those were currently investigated by the American College of Radiology Imaging Network (ACRIN) National CTC Trial (Hara et al. 2011). The polyp detection rate was comparable among PEG, NaP, and magnesium citrate, although NaP had the highest patient compliance and the least residual stool (Hara et al. 2011).

Despite the endorsement as an acceptable option for colorectal cancer screening, the governmental health care system recently decide not to cover CTC for screening purpose in the United States (Heiken 2009; Garg and Ahnen 2010). The reasons for which include radiation exposure, false-negative rates for smaller polyps, the discovery of extracolonic findings leading to excess RAIs, variability in performance, lack of targeted studies, and absence of clear definitions of expertise and certification (Garg and Ahnen 2010). Furthermore, an evident limitation of CTC screening is that so far there is no study demonstrating the efficacy of CTC in reducing the CRC incidence and mortality (Davila et al. 2006).

However, given the lesser invasive nature and having lesser perceived discomfort compared to colonoscopy, CTC may improve compliance rate in CRC screening and provide an important role as an adjunctive screening modality, particularly in the elderly community (McFarland et al. 2009; Heresbach et al. 2011).

Conclusions

It must be reminded that the ideal purpose of screening is to detect and eradicate precancerous or cancerous diseases, thereby that can reduce cancer-related mortality in asymptomatic individuals. Current concepts and evidences support that colonoscopy is the most feasible examination for CRC screening at any ages of patients. Screening colonoscopy in the elderly patients should be performed after careful consideration for indication with full informed consent with regard to potential benefits and risks relative to procedure. Furthermore, health care providers should be aware that increasing screening rates may lead to increase in false-positive results, cancer overdiagnosis, morbidity and mortality from screening procedure and/or downstream treatments, and monetary burden on both patients and health care system.

References

Allison JE, Tekawa IS et al (1996) A comparison of fecal occult-blood tests for colorectal-cancer screening. N Engl J Med 334(3):155–159

Arora A, Singh P (2004) Colonoscopy in patients 80 years of age and older is safe, with high success rate and diagnostic yield. Gastrointest Endosc 60(3):408–413

Belsey J, Epstein O et al (2007) Systematic review: oral bowel preparation for colonoscopy. Aliment Pharmacol Ther 25(4):373–384

Cohen LB (2010) Split dosing of bowel preparations for colonoscopy: an analysis of its efficacy, safety, and tolerability. Gastrointest Endosc 72(2):406–412

Curran MP, Plosker GL (2004) Oral sodium phosphate solution: a review of its use as a colorectal cleanser. Drugs 64(15):1697–1714

Davila RE, Rajan E et al (2006) ASGE guideline: colorectal cancer screening and surveillance. Gastrointest Endosc 63(4):546–557

Day LW, Kwon A et al (2011a) Adverse events in older patients undergoing colonoscopy: a systematic review and meta-analysis. Gastrointest Endosc 74(4):885–896

Day LW, Walter LC et al (2011b) Colorectal cancer screening and surveillance in the elderly patient. Am J Gastroenterol 106(7):1197–1206

de Haan MC, van Gelder RE et al (2011) Diagnostic value of CT-colonography as compared to colonoscopy in an asymptomatic screening population: a meta-analysis. Eur Radiol 21(8):1747–1763

El Sayed AM, Kanafani ZA et al (2003) A randomized single-blind trial of whole versus split-dose polyethylene glycol-electrolyte solution for colonoscopy preparation. Gastrointest Endosc 58(1):36–40

Garg S, Ahnen DJ (2010) Is computed tomographic colonography being held to a higher standard? Ann Intern Med 152(3):178–181

Goodwin JS, Singh A et al (2011) Overuse of screening colonoscopy in the Medicare population. Arch Intern Med 171(15):1335–1343

Greenberg PD, Bertario L et al (2000) A prospective multicenter evaluation of new fecal occult blood tests in patients undergoing colonoscopy. Am J Gastroenterol 95(5):1331–1338

Hara AK, Kuo MD et al (2011) National CT colonography trial (ACRIN 6664): comparison of three full-laxative bowel preparations in more than 2500 average-risk patients. AJR Am J Roentgenol 196(5):1076–1082

Harada Y, Hirasawa D et al (2009) Impact of a transparent hood on the performance of total colonoscopy: a randomized controlled trial. Gastrointest Endosc 69(3 Pt 2):637–644

Hardcastle JD, Chamberlain JO et al (1996) Randomised controlled trial of faecal-occult-blood screening for colorectal cancer. Lancet 348(9040):1472–1477

Heiken JP (2009) CT colonography screening: ready for prime time? Cancer Imaging 9(Spec No A):S59–S62

Heresbach D, Djabbari M et al (2011) Accuracy of computed tomographic colonography in a nationwide multicentre trial, and its relation to radiologist expertise. Gut 60(5):658–665

Horiuchi A, Nakayama Y et al (2008) Propofol sedation for endoscopic procedures in patients 90 years of age and older. Digestion 78(1):20–23

Juluri R, Eckert G et al (2011) Polyethylene glycol vs. sodium phosphate for bowel preparation: a treatment arm meta-analysis of randomized controlled trials. BMC Gastroenterol 11:38

Karajeh MA, Sanders DS et al (2006) Colonoscopy in elderly people is a safe procedure with a high diagnostic yield: a prospective comparative study of 2000 patients. Endoscopy 38(3):226–230

Keedy AW, Yee J et al (2011) Reduced cathartic bowel preparation for CT colonography: prospective comparison of 2-L polyethylene glycol and magnesium citrate. Radiology 261(1):156–164

Kistler CE, Kirby KA et al (2011) Long-term outcomes following positive fecal occult blood test results in older adults: benefits and burdens. Arch Intern Med 171(15):1344–1351

Ko CW, Sonnenberg A (2005) Comparing risks and benefits of colorectal cancer screening in elderly patients. Gastroenterology 129(4):1163–1170

Kondo S, Yamaji Y et al (2007) A randomized controlled trial evaluating the usefulness of a transparent hood attached to the tip of the colonoscope. Am J Gastroenterol 102(1):75–81

Kronborg O, Fenger C et al (1996) Randomised study of screening for colorectal cancer with faecal-occult-blood test. Lancet 348(9040):1467–1471

Lawrance IC, Willert RP et al (2011) Bowel cleansing for colonoscopy: prospective randomized assessment of efficacy and of induced mucosal abnormality with three preparation agents. Endoscopy 43(5):412–418

Lee SH, Chung IK et al (2008) An adequate level of training for technical competence in screening and diagnostic colonoscopy: a prospective multicenter evaluation of the learning curve. Gastrointest Endosc 67(4):683–689

Lichtenstein GR, Cohen LB et al (2007) Review article: Bowel preparation for colonoscopy – the importance of adequate hydration. Aliment Pharmacol Ther 26(5):633–641

Lin OS, Kozarek RA et al (2006) Screening colonoscopy in very elderly patients: prevalence of neoplasia and estimated impact on life expectancy. JAMA 295(20):2357–2365

Lukens FJ, Loeb DS et al (2002) Colonoscopy in octogenarians: a prospective outpatient study. Am J Gastroenterol 97(7):1722–1725

Macari M, Nevsky G et al (2011) CT colonography in senior versus nonsenior patients: extracolonic findings, recommendations for additional imaging, and polyp prevalence. Radiology 259(3):767–774

Mandel JS, Bond JH et al (1993) Reducing mortality from colorectal cancer by screening for fecal occult blood. Minnesota Colon Cancer Control Study. N Engl J Med 328(19):1365–1371

McFarland EG, Fletcher JG et al (2009) ACR Colon Cancer Committee white paper: status of CT colonography 2009. J Am Coll Radiol 6(11):756–772 e.4

Nelson DB, McQuaid KR et al (2002) Procedural success and complications of large-scale screening colonoscopy. Gastrointest Endosc 55(3):307–314

Schmilovitz-Weiss H, Weiss A et al (2007) Predictors of failed colonoscopy in nonagenarians: a single-center experience. J Clin Gastroenterol 41(4):388–393

Seinela L, Pehkonen E et al (2003) Bowel preparation for colonoscopy in very old patients: a randomized prospective trial comparing oral sodium phosphate and polyethylene glycol electrolyte lavage solution. Scand J Gastroenterol 38(2):216–220

Takeuchi Y, Inoue T et al (2010) Surveillance colonoscopy using a transparent hood and image-enhanced endoscopy. Dig Endosc 22(Suppl 1):S47–S53

Thomson A, Naidoo P et al (1996) Bowel preparation for colonoscopy: a randomized prospective trail comparing sodium phosphate and polyethylene glycol in a predominantly elderly population. J Gastroenterol Hepatol 11(2):103–107

Tsutsumi S, Fukushima H et al (2007) Feasibility of colonoscopy in patients 80 years of age and older. Hepatogastroenterology 54(79):1959–1961

US Preventive Services Task Force (2008) Screening for colorectal cancer: U.S. Preventive Services Task Force recommendation statement. Ann Intern Med 149(9):627–637

Walter LC, Covinsky KE (2001) Cancer screening in elderly patients: a framework for individualized decision making. JAMA 285(21):2750–2756

Wexner SD, Beck DE et al (2006) A consensus document on bowel preparation before colonoscopy: prepared by a task force from the American Society of Colon and Rectal Surgeons (ASCRS), the American Society for Gastrointestinal Endoscopy (ASGE), and the Society of American Gastrointestinal and Endoscopic Surgeons (SAGES). Gastrointest Endosc 63(7):894–909

Risk Stratification for Elderly Surgery

3

Emile Chung-Hou Woo and Kok-Yang Tan

Take Home Pearls

- Pre operative risk stratification in the elderly patient is important not only to predict mortality and morbidity but also to predict return to baseline function.
- These processes also facilitate targeted interventions prior to surgery.
- There are both medical and surgical assessment tools that are useful.
- Geriatric assessment tools are equally important in elderly surgical patients and may identify patients with a reduced functional reserve which conventional tools may miss.
- Due to heterogeneity, morbidities are better quantified rather than described.
- Outcome measures should not only include morbidity and mortality but also return to functional baseline.

E.C.-H. Woo, B.Sc. (Pharm)., M.D., FRCSC, FACS (✉)
Department of Surgery,
University of British Columbia,
Vancouver, Canada
e-mail: emile.woo@gmail.com

K.-Y. Tan, MBBS(Melb), MMed(Surg), FRCS, FAMS
Department of General Surgery,
Khoo Teck Puat Hospital,
Singapore, Singapore
e-mail: kokyangtan@gmail.com

K.-Y. Tan (ed.), *Colorectal Cancer in the Elderly*,
DOI 10.1007/978-3-642-29883-7_3, © Springer-Verlag Berlin Heidelberg 2013

3.1   Introduction

Preoperative risk stratification for the elderly is extremely important and serves three functions:

1. Assist in the decision to offer surgery or not
2. Assist in the perioperative management of the patient
3. Assist in presenting the patient with adequate information for informed consent

Of particular importance, and perhaps uniquely in the geriatric population, the decision to choose between a surgical intervention or not can be a complex process. Typically, when a patient is diagnosed with a malignancy that is resectable, surgery generally follows. However, in the geriatric population, one must consider whether the cure, i.e., surgical intervention to extend life, will compete with the patient's expectation with regard to quality of life. If surgery can extend life but comes with a high risk of mortality and morbidity and result in a patient unlikely returning to their baseline function, then, is he or she better served by foregoing surgery and an extended but low-quality lifespan and instead choose to live a shorter lifespan but with a better quality of life? One must ask whether an otherwise high-functioning patient would desire surgery if there is a substantial risk that he or she will become bed bound or lose their independence permanently.

The second reason for the need for risk stratification is to allow for better perioperative management of the patient that chooses to undergo surgery. This allows recognition of specific physiological problems that may be better optimized preoperatively or require close postoperative monitoring. In the elderly patient, this is no simple task as a significant number of patients will present with more than one comorbidity and may be on multiple medications that will impact perioperative care. Coupled with age-related decreases in functional reserves, a thorough and holistic risk analysis can be a daunting task.

It also goes without saying that in order to provide patients with proper informed consent, the surgical risks and their likelihoods is a very important area of concern that requires adequate discussion prior to surgery. Moreover, the impact on the patient's quality of life will need to be discussed in detail both for decision making and for the patient to make adequate plans for long-term postoperative care.

Lastly, one should also keep in mind the goals of treatment. It is certainly obvious that, if the patient has decided on surgery for treatment, the goals are to maximize the therapeutic benefit of the intervention leading to cure and to minimize perioperative morbidity and mortality. However, just as important, as alluded to previously, is for the geriatric patient to return to baseline function. In some ways, this goal is even more difficult than the others. As such, unique to geriatric surgery, is the need to document a patient's baseline function, have a plan to return to this baseline, and measure if this occurs postoperatively.

3.2   General Risk Scoring Systems

A number of general risk scoring systems are in common use today. These are either physiological-based or organ system-specific systems that deal with perioperative morbidity and mortality.

Table 3.1 American Society of Anesthesiologists Physical Status classification system

ASA status	Criteria
1	A normal healthy patient
2	A patient with mild systemic disease
3	A patient with severe systemic disease
4	A patient with severe systemic disease that is a constant threat to life
5	A moribund patient who is not expected to survive without the operation
6	A declared brain-dead patient whose organs are being removed for donor purposes

3.2.1   ASA Physical Status Scoring System

In 1941, the American Society of Anesthetists made the first attempt by any medical specialty to risk stratify patients in the form of the ASA physical status classification system (Table 3.1). A three-person committee was tasked to develop a system to collect and tabulate anesthetic data. It is thus useful for record keeping and for statistical analyses looking at perioperative data. This widely used classification system determines risk solely on the basis of a patient's preoperative history and is relatively easy to use.

Of note is that the ASA classification was not designed as a tool to predict postoperative morbidity or mortality. There is no attempt to quantify the risk. As such, it is a relatively crude instrument for the analysis of operative risk. However, there have been studies that have sought to validate the ASA scoring system and have shown that the ASA score does correlate with outcomes such as unplanned ICU admissions, cardiopulmonary adverse events, and prolonged hospital stay. As such, it is still widely used by anesthetists for perioperative planning.

In the context of geriatric surgery, it is important to note that age is not a criteria along with other important variables such as type of surgery, degree of weight loss, etc. As well, it is to be noted that this scoring system uses subjective measures as opposed to objective, measured indicators.

3.2.2   Goldman and Detsky Index

In an attempt to better determine and quantify risk, Goldman, in 1977, developed a risk assessment tool using nine variables to determine cardiac risk for noncardiac surgery patients (Goldman et al. 1977). Each variable is assigned a point value and a patient's risk is determined based on the overall score (Table 3.2). The highest possible score in this system is 53. Based on this scoring scheme, patients can be classified into four distinct categories of risks (Table 3.3). His tool was derived retrospectively using a database of 1,001 patients.

This multifactorial tool certainly was a step forward from the ASA scoring system as it is an objective scale that is designed to give a predicted score. However, it only is designed to predict the possibility of a cardiovascular event and therefore

Table 3.2 Goldman's multi-factorial index

Variable	Points
History	
Myocardial infarction within 6 months	10
Age over 70	5
Physical examination	
S-3 or jugular venous distension	11
Important aortic stenosis	3
Electrocardiogram	
Rhythm other than sinus or sinus plus APBs on last preoperative ECG	7
More than 5 premature ventricular beats per minute at any time preoperatively	7
Poor general medical status – O_2 pressure <60 mmHg, CO_2 pressure >50 mmHg, Serum K+<3 mmol/L, Serum HCO_3 <20 mmol/L, serum urea>18 mmol/L, serum creatinine>260 mmol/L, AST abnormal, signs of chronic liver disease, and/or bedridden from noncardiac causes	3
Intraperitoneal, intrathoracic, or aortic surgery	3
Emergency operation	4

Table 3.3 Risk of cardiac complications based on Goldman's score

Total score	Risk of cardiac complications (%)
0–5	1
6–12	7
13–25	14
26–53	78

will under evaluate the total mortality and morbidity risk. As well, the authors did not subsequently perform hypothesis testing after the score was developed. It is still a useful tool given the fact that cardiovascular problems are the most common comorbidity encountered in the geriatric population.

In 1986, Detsky further refined Goldman's original system by adding newer criteria such as pulmonary edema (Detsky et al. 1986a) (Table 3.4). As well, a further attempt was made to incorporate the type of surgery that the patient was to undergo into the risk calculation. The surgical categories were major vascular surgery, orthopedic, intrathoracic/intraperitoneal, and minor surgery. This generated a pretest probability ranging from 1.6% to 13.6%. Then, a nomogram was used in conjunction with the modified multifactorial index to generate a posttest probability of a severe cardiac complication. Both the original Goldman index and Detsky index continue to be used, and web-based calculators are easily found and can be quickly used to calculate both scores and predicted risk of complications.

Table 3.4 Detsky modified multifactorial index

Variables	Points
Coronary artery disease	
1. Myocardial infarction <6 months	10
2. Myocardial infarction >6 months	5
Canadian Cardiovascular Society Angina	
1. Class 3	10
2. Class 4	20
3. Unstable angina within 3 months	5
Valvular disease: suspected critical aortic stenosis	20
Arrhythmias	
1. Sinus plus atrial premature beats or rhythm other than sinus on last preoperative ECG	5
2. More than 5 ventricular premature beats at any time prior to surgery	5
Poor general medical status: O_2 pressure <60 mmHg, CO_2 pressure >50 mmHg, Serum K+<3 mmol/L, Serum HCO_3 <20 mmol/L, serum urea >18 mmol/L, serum creatinine >260 mmol/L, AST abnormal, signs of chronic liver disease, and/or bedridden from noncardiac causes	5
Age over 70 years	5
Emergency operation	10

3.2.3   American College of Cardiology/American Heart Association Guidelines

Subsequently, the American College of Cardiology and the American Heart Association developed a joint guideline for preoperative cardiovascular evaluation for noncardiac surgery. The latest guideline was updated 2007 (Fleisher et al. 2007) and is available for download at http://content.onlinejacc.org/cgi/content/full/50/17/e159. Although the algorithm is not strictly a tool to calculate risk, it is a useful guide with respect to determining which patients may benefit or require further pre-optimization. One of the strengths of the tool is that that there is an emphasis on minimizing unnecessary procedures and tests, which would undoubtedly lead to a longer preoperative course.

3.2.4   POSSUM Scoring

Coming out of the need to develop a useful surgical audit tool to compare performance across hospitals, Copland in 1991 published a paper wherein they performed a multivariable analysis to determine independent risk factors affecting morbidity and mortality (Copeland et al. 1991). This led to the development of the Physiological and Operative Severity Score for the enUmeration of Mortality and morbidity (POSSUM). The score comprises 12 preoperative and 6 intraoperative variables to predict for both mortality and morbidity (Table 3.5). Thus, a physiologic score based on the patient's preoperative risk factors is combined with six intraoperative findings to give a more comprehensive predictor. Further analysis of this tool in the literature noted that the POSSUM score tended to overpredict mortality in low-risk patients.

Subsequently, Prytherch and colleagues developed a modification of the score known as the (Portsmouth) P-POSSUM (Prytherch et al. 1998). This score was developed in response to the short coming of overpredicting low-risk patient's mortality and was based on the same data set used for the original POSSUM score. However, the P-POSSUM score tends to underestimate the risk in both the elderly and in emergency surgeries. Used together, the POSSUM score can be used for morbidity and the P-POSSUM is then used for mortality. Both of these scores have been validated as a tool for the use in general surgery and are widely used in the western world.

A further refinement to the POSSUM score is the Cr-POSSUM score (Table 3.6) that is specifically designed for use in colorectal surgery (Tekkis et al. 2004). Of the three, the Cr-POSSUM appears to predict mortality better than both of the above. Lastly, in 2010, Tran developed the E-POSSUM score that is further defined for use in the elderly population undergoing colorectal surgery (Tran et al. 2010). It has yet to be externally validated.

3.3   Geriatric Risk Assessment

What is of utmost importance with regard to the geriatric patient is that none of these above risk stratification systems deal with what Bernard Isaacs termed "the giants of geriatrics": immobility, instability, incontinence, and cognitive impairment (Issacs 1997). Immobility of course is a big issue with regard to postoperative mobilization and the prevention of such conditions such as venous thromboembolism and pneumonia. Instability, of course, can lead to falls which again will cause other comorbidities such as fractures and, one of the most concerning problems, which is head trauma. Incontinence places the patient at risk of soilage and cross-contamination. And lastly, cognitive impairment is one of the biggest risks for postoperative confusion and delirium.

3.3.1   Charlson Weighted Comorbidity Index

It is therefore fitting to look toward the geriatric literature to better understand risk assessment in the geriatric population. One risk assessment tool commonly used in the geriatric population is the Charlson weighted comorbidity index (Charlson et al. 1987). This tool was initially developed to assess long-term mortality in this population of patients. However, subsequently, it has been used to predict outcomes for acute

Table 3.5 POSSUM scoring and formula for predicted morbidity and mortality

	1	2	4	8
POSSUM physiological score				
Age	<60	61–70	>71	
Cardiac + CXR	No failure	Diuretic, digoxin, antianginal/hypertensive	Dyspnea on exertion, moderate COPD	Resting dyspnea, RR>30/min, fibrosis, consolidation
Systolic BP	110–130	131–170 or 100–109	>171 or 90–99	<90
Heart rate/min	50–80	81–100 or 40–49	101–120	>121 or <40
GCS	15	12–14	9–11	<8
Hb	13–16	11.5–12.9 or 16.1–17.0	10.0–11.4 or 17.1–18.0	<9.9 or >18.1
WBC	4–10	10.1–20.0 or 3.1–4.0	>20.1 or <3.0	>15.1
Urea	<7.5	7.6–10.0	10.1–15.0	>15.1
Sodium	>136	131–135	126–130	<125
Potassium	3.5–5.0	3.2–3.4 or 5.1–5.3	2.9–3.1 or 5.4–5.9	<2.8 or >6.0
ECG	Normal		Atria fibrillation (rate 60–90/min)	Any abnormal rhythm, >5 ectopics/min, Q waves, ST/T wave changes
POSSUM operative severity score				
Severity score	Minor	Moderate (colectomies)	Major (APR)	Major +
Multiple procedures	1		2	>2
Blood loss (mls)	<100	101–500	501–999	>999
Contamination	None	Minor (serous)	Local pus	Free bowel content, pus or blood
Presence of Ca	None	Primary	Nodal mets	Distant mets
Mode of surgery	Elective		Urgent	Emergency (immediate <2 h)

$x = (0.16 \times \text{physiologic score}) + (0.19 \times \text{operative score}) - 5.91$
Predicted morbidity rate $= 1/(1 + e^{(-x)})$
$y = (0.13 \times \text{physiologic score}) + (0.16 \times \text{operative score}) - 7.04$
Predicted mortality rate $= 1/(1 + e^{(-y)})$

Table 3.6 Colorectal POSSUM

	1	2	3	4	8
Physiological parameters					
Age	<61	–	61–70	71–80	>80
Cardiac failure	No/mild	Moderate	Severe	–	–
Systolic BP (mmHg)	100–170	>171 or 90–99	<89	–	–
Heart rate (beats/min)	40–100	101–120	>121 or <39	–	–
Hb level (g/dL)	13–16	10–12.9 or 16.1–18	<9.9 or >18.1	–	–
Urea level	<10	10.1–15	>15	–	–
Operative parameters					
Operation type	Minor	–	Intermediate	Major	Complex major
Peritoneal contamination	None/serous fluid	Local pus	Free bowel content, pus or blood	–	–
Malignancy status	No cancer/dukes A or B	Dukes C	Dukes D	–	–
Urgency	Elective	–	Urgent	–	Emergency (<2 h)

Table 3.7 Weighted index of comorbidity from Charlson comorbidity index

Comorbidity condition	Assigned weighted index
Acquired immune deficiency syndrome (AIDS)	6
Metastatic solid malignancy	6
Liver disease – moderate or severe	3
Malignant lymphoma	2
Leukemia	2
Any malignancy	2
Diabetes with end organ damage	2
Renal disease – moderate or severe	2
Hemiplegia	2
Diabetes	1
Liver disease – mild	1
Ulcer disease	1
Connective tissue disease	1
Chronic pulmonary disease	1
Dementia	1
Cerebrovascular disease	1
Peripheral vascular disease	1
Congestive heart failure	1
Myocardial infarction	1

medical events such as a cerebral vascular accident. Furthermore, it has been adapted for use in the surgical arena in such diverse conditions such as transplantation, mesenteric ischemia, and also perforated diverticular disease. In the realm of colorectal surgery in particular, a recent study found that a comorbidity score higher than 5 predicted for a 5 times higher risk of morbidity.

The scale itself consists of a number of comorbidities that are given a weighted value (Table 3.7). The aggregate score thus gives the clinician a tool to quantify the burden of disease. Of note is that this is primarily a geriatrician's tool and not a surgeon's tool.

3.3.2   Frailty

A more recent and emerging concept is that of frailty. Frailty is fast becoming as recognized as another "giant" of geriatrics as the term tries to capture the overall patient's hardiness and resilience to injury (Crome and Lally 2011). The core concepts of frailty are not in doubt, and there is consensus that frailty is a condition in which patients have impairments in multiple, interrelated systems that lead to increased vulnerability to physiological challenges and stressors. There is a loss of resiliency due to decreased functional reserves. What is interesting in regard to this concept is that it is not necessarily comorbidity based. There are patients who have multiple comorbidities and are not frail, but conversely, there are patients who have no comorbidities but are frail.

Where there is a lack of consensus is how frailty should be defined. In the literature, the most commonly cited definitions are by Fried and Rockwood. Fried's model (Fried et al. 2001) is based on the assessment of five physical indicators: weight loss, walking speed, grip strength, physical activity, and exhaustion (Table 3.8). A finding of impairment in three or more categories meets the diagnosis of frailty. The scale has been shown to predict for falls, disability, hospital admission, and mortality. Most recently, our institution has shown that that in patients who meet the criteria for frailty, the odds ratio related to postoperative major complications was fourfold (4.083 [CI 1.433–11.638]) (Tan et al. 2011). A recent study by Makary using the Fried criteria found that it predicted for postoperative complications, length of stay, as well as discharge from hospital into a facility (Makary et al. 2010).

Some drawbacks to the Fried model are that it is difficult to apply to patients who are acutely ill and that it lacks direct measurement of mental health and psychosocial status.

Rockwood's model proposes that the risk of becoming frail is related to the development of certain deficits. As such, as more and more deficits accumulate, the greater the risk of frailty will be. However, the model has yet to be fully accepted in the clinical setting and has not been tested in the surgical literature (Rockwood et al. 2005).

3.3.3 Baseline Function

The various standard systems noted previously reflect the typical risk stratification tools that measure the risk of mortality and perioperative complications. However, one of the biggest critiques of the state of geriatric surgery is that outcomes studies are missing the mark and that these outcome measures of morbidity and mortality, though extremely useful, do not address possibly the biggest concern of the geriatric population: what will be the quality of life after surgery? Surgeons are adept at looking into morbidity and mortality rates to best contemplate whether a surgical intervention is worthwhile and can compare it to the natural history of the disease as well as the possibility of cure based on the tumor type and surgical procedure. What is not commonly addressed both by surgeons and the literature is what is the rate of return to baseline function and, hence, quality of life after surgical intervention. There is a need to remind caregivers that health is not merely absence of disease or cancer in this case, but the state of complete physical, mental, and social well-being. As well, the affect on postoperative function can have a direct impact on survival that is separate from any tumor stage considerations.

Currently, there is a dearth of tools and knowledge as to the affect that colorectal rectal surgery has on quality of life and return to baseline function. At the minimum, any surgical unit that performs geriatric surgery should consider using a tool such as Barthel's activities of daily living index (Table 3.9) to use as a baseline score and then follow this out postoperatively and to collect this data prospectively to better understand and quantify the impact that surgery has on baseline function.

Table 3.8 Criteria for definition of frailty

Components	Details of criteria			Satisfy criteria
Gender	Male	Female		
Weight loss	Greater than 10 lbs or 5% weight loss in the last 1 year			Yes/no
15 – foot walk time	More than or equal to 7 s	Height less than or equal to 159 cm	More than or equal to 7 s	Yes/no
	More than or equal to 6 s	Height more than 159 cm	More than or equal to 6 s	
Grip strength	BMI less than or equal to 24	BMI less than or equal to 23	Less than or equal to 17	Yes/no
	BMI 24.1–26	BMI 23.1–26	Less than or equal to 17.3	
	BMI 26.1–28	BMI 26.1–28	Less than or equal to 18	
	BMI more than 28	BMI more than 29	Less than or equal to 21	
Physical activity (MLTA)	Less than 383 kcal/week	Less than 270 kcal/week		Yes/no
Exhaustion	A score of 2 or 3 on either of the question on CES – D below:			Yes/no
	How often in the last week did you feel this way?			
	1. I felt that everything I did was an effort			
	2. I could not get going			
	Score: 0 = 1 day, 1 = 1–2 days, 2 = 3–4 days, 3 = more than 4 days			

One is *frail* having satisfied three or more of above criteria (i.e., three or more "Yes")

Table 3.9 Modified Barthel's index

Components	Unable to perform task	Attempts task but unsafe	Moderate help required	Minimal help required	Fully Independent
Personal hygiene	0	1	3	4	5
Bathing self	0	1	3	4	5
Feeding	0	2	5	8	10
Toileting	0	2	5	8	10
Stair climbing	0	2	5	8	10
Dressing	0	2	5	8	10
Bowel control	0	2	5	8	10
Bladder control	0	2	5	8	10
Ambulation	0	3	8	12	15
(wheelchair)	0	1	3	4	5
Chair-bed transfer	0	3	8	12	15
Total score		/100			

This will continue to be an ever expanding area of inquiry and concern. The aim, of course, is to be able to nurture patients back to their baseline function should they decide on surgery.

3.3.4 Comprehensive Geriatric Assessment

The above three parameters form part of a comprehensive assessment which has potential implications that are wider than surgical risk assessment alone and thus have been mentioned in other chapters in this book as well.

Conclusion

With the myriad of tools that have been developed, colorectal surgeons should become familiarized with at least one physiological scoring system and one that looks at frailty. At this time, the best tools available appear to be the Cr-POSSUM score as well as Fried's frailty index. Using a combination of these tools will allow the clinician to better consider the appropriateness of surgery for each individual patient and also use this information to better allow the patient to give informed consent.

An increasing emphasis needs to be placed on the patient's return to baseline function. We need to expand our definition of surgical success not only on tumor cure and absence of morbidity and mortality, but also on the patient's ability to return to their prior level of function. For patients who are undergoing surgery, Barthel's index should be used to document baseline function and subsequently allow for postoperative goal setting as well as quality assurance. As hinted above, having a geriatrician as an active part of the team is invaluable and the use of the Charlson index can be added.

As the geriatric population increases, the need for more colorectal surgery will also increase and more and better tools will be required to better help select which patients will benefit from surgery. The need though is for better tools to predict not just morbidity or mortality, but to also predict for quality of life and the ability of the patient to return to baseline function. A further challenge is for the development of effective tools to mitigate and/or alleviate the problem of frailty. As such, all colorectal units have an obligation to prospectively collect and routinely analyze their data to develop newer and better protocols to treat the elderly patient with colorectal cancer.

References

Saklad M (1941) Grading of Patients for Surgical Parodures. Anesthesioloygy 2(3);272–280

Charlson ME, Pompei P, Ales KL, MacKenzie CR (1987) A new method of classifying prognostic comorbidity in longitudinal studies: development and validation. J Chronic Dis 40(5):373–383

Copeland GP, Jones D, Walters M (1991) POSSUM: a scoring system for surgical audit. Br J Surg 78(3):355–360

Crome P, Lally F (2011) Frailty: joining the giants. Can Med Assoc J 183(8):889–890

Detsky AS, Abrams HB, Forbath N, Scott JG, Hilliard JR (1986a) Cardiac assessment for patients undergoing non cardiac surgery: a multifactorial clinical risk index. Arch Intern Med 146: 2131–2134

Detsky A, Abrams HB, McLaughlin JR, Drucker DJ, Sasson Z, Johnston N, Scott JG, Forbath N, Hilliard JR (1986b) Predicting cardiac complications in patients undergoing non-cardiac surgery. J Gen Intern Med 1(4):211–219

Fleisher LA et al (2007) ACC/AHA 2007 guidelines on perioperative cardiovascular evaluation for noncardiac surgery: a report of the American College of Cardiology/American Heart Association Task Force on Practice Guidelines. J Am Coll Cardiol 50:e159–e242

Fried LP, Tangen CM, Walston J, Newman AB, Hirsch C, Gottdiener J et al (2001) Frailty in older adults: evidence for a pheno- type. J Gerontol A Biol Sci Med Sci 56(3):M146–M156

Goldman L, Caldera DL, Nussbaum SR, Southwick FS, Krogstad D, Murray B, Burke DS, O'Malley TA, Goroll AH, Caplan CH, Nolan J, Carabello B, Slatter EE (1977) Multifactorial index of cardiac risk in noncardiac surgical procedures. N Engl J Med 297(16):845–850

Issacs B (1997) The challenge of geriatric medicine. Oxford University Press, Oxford

Makary MA, Segev DL, Pronovost PJ, Syin D, Bandeen-Roche K, Patel P, Takenaga R, Devgan L, Holzmueller CG, Tian J, Fried P (2010) Frailty as a predictor of surgical outcomes of older patients. J Am Coll Surg 39:412–423

Prytherch DR, Whitely MS, Weaver PC, Prout WG, Powell SJ (1998) POSSUM and Portsmouth POSSUM for predicting mortality. Br J Surg 85(9):1217–1220

Rockwood K, Song X, MacKnight C et al (2005) A global clinical measure of fitness and frailty in elderly people. Can Med Assoc J 173:489–495

Tan KY, Kawamura YJ, Tokomitsu A, Tang T (2011) Assessment for frailty is useful for predicting morbidity in elderly patients undergoing colorectal cancer resection whose comorbidities are already optimized. Am J Surg [Epub ahead of print]

Tekkis PP, Prytherch DR, Kocher HM, Senapati A, Poloniecki JD, Stamatakis JD, Windsor AC (2004) Development of a dedicated risk-adjustment scoring system for colorectal surgery (colorectal POSSUM). Br J Surg 91(9):1174–1182

Tran BLP, du Montcel ST, Duron JJ, Levard H, Suc B, Descottes B, Desrousseaux B, Hay JM (2010) Elderly POSSUM, a dedicated score for prediction of mortality and morbidity after major colorectal surgery in older patients. Br J Surg 97(3):296–403

Rational Approach to Cancer in the Elderly

4

Frédérique Retornaz, Maud Cécile, and Howard Bergman

Take Home Pearls

- Colorectal cancer is a frequent and potentially curable disease (when localized) in the elderly.
- Decision making in the elderly is complex due to the underlying health status that can interfere with the management from diagnosis to treatment.
- Preserving the quality of life and autonomy are more important to consider in this population rather than increased survival alone. However, physicians tend to underestimate life expectancy that will lead to suboptimal management.
- Some form of geriatric assessment done at the time of diagnosis may help the physician in their decision making.

F. Retornaz, M.D., Ph.D. (✉)
Unité de coordination en oncogériatrie (UCOG),
Centre Gérontologique Départemental,
1 rue Elzéard Rougier, 13012 Marseille, France

EA3279. Evaluation des Systèmes de Soins – Santé Perçue,
Université de la Méditerranée, 27 bd Jean Moulin, 13006 Marseille, France
e-mail: fretornaz.cgd13@e-santepaca.fr

M. Cécile, M.D.
Unité pilote de coordination en oncogériatrie (UPCOG), Institut Paoli Calmettes,
232 Bd Sainte Marguerite, 13273 Marseille, cedex 9, France
e-mail: cecilem@marseille.fnclcc.fr

H. Bergman, M.D.
Division of Geriatric Medicine, Jewish General Hospital,
3755 Côte Ste-Catherine, Montreal, QC, Canada H3T 1E2

Solidage Research Group on Integrated Services for Older Persons,
Centre for Clinical Epidemiology and Community Studies, Jewish General Hospital,
3755 Côte Ste-Catherine, Montreal, QC, Canada H3T 1E2
e-mail: howard.bergman@mcgill.ca

K.-Y. Tan (ed.), *Colorectal Cancer in the Elderly*,
DOI 10.1007/978-3-642-29883-7_4, © Springer-Verlag Berlin Heidelberg 2013

4.1 Introduction

The incidence and mortality of cancer increase with age (Yancik and Ries 2000). Over 60% of cancers and more than 70% of cancer deaths occur in people over 65. The risk of cancer in this age group is 11 times higher than in people under 65. Thus, two-thirds of tumors of the colon, rectum, stomach, pancreas, prostate, and urinary tract affect patients older than 65. Colorectal cancer is the second cause of death among people over 65 (Aouba et al. 2007). Due to the aging population and the increased cancer incidence due to age, clinicians should expect that they will have to care for an ever growing number of elderly cancer patients.

4.2 Specific to Colorectal Cancer in the Elderly

4.2.1 Epidemiological Data

The number of new cancer cases (all types) almost doubled between 1980 and 2005 (170,000–320,000), and over 45% of these cancers were diagnosed in the population of patients aged 70 and over. Colorectal cancer is a disease of the elderly. The average age at diagnosis is 70 for men and 73 for women. Colorectal cancers are the third cause in terms of incidence and the second cause in terms of mortality in people aged over 65. Over 75% of deaths from colorectal cancers involve patients over 70.

4.2.2 Why Treat Elderly Patients with Colorectal Cancer?

Data from the National Institute of Statistics and Economic Studies (INSEE) show that overall life expectancy has increased. According to estimates in France, in 2020, life expectancy at birth will be 78.1 years for men and 86.4 years for women (http://www.iinsee.fr). In 2050, it will be 82.2 years for men and 90.4 years for women. In 2050, one out of every three will have lived 60 or more years. In 1991, life expectancy was 73 years for men and 81.1 years for women. Between 1981 and 1991, life expectancy without disability increased by 3 years for men and by 2.6 years for women. All these data indicate the need for concerted and optimal management of cancer in the elderly (Aparicio et al. 2005). Yet it is often the idea of a shortened life expectancy that leads doctors and family not to propose optimal management. Montaigne said, "Age imprints more wrinkles in the mind than it does on the face." Are we really "too old" at age 70? A person who has reached that age still has an additional life expectancy estimated overall to 14.2 years. An 80-year life expectancy has an additional 7.7 years; an 85-year expectancy, an additional 5.4 years. Beyond these theoretical figures, it should be noted that three-quarters of the population over the age of 85 lives independently at home, without any major physiological or psychological impairment.

The main question is whether newly diagnosed elderly cancer patients will suffer from the cancer, in particular those who have slow-growing cancers such as prostate, breast, and kidney. The treatment decision is based more on the state of the patient's underlying health than on the cancer itself. We should not treat slowly evolving tumors that will never become symptomatic in patients whose life expectancy is already limited by comorbidities or impaired functional status. In the case of colorectal cancer, most patients – except those with a very short life expectancy (less than 6 months) – will suffer from complications that include anemia, obstruction, perforation, metastasis, and others. In most cases, the life expectancy of an elderly patient is often underestimated by the family and the physician. Consequently, too often do patients come to us with advanced stages or even with metastases, even though a potentially curative treatment would have been possible. Treatment options had been rejected a few months or years earlier because the cancer was not considered then to be an immediate threat to the patient's survival. To underestimate the potential impact of cancer and life expectancy can expose an elderly patient to a high risk of loss of autonomy and of deterioration in the quality of life that could have been preserved longer had we decided to control the tumor at diagnosis. Finding the right balance between cancer burden and life expectancy remains the main priority of oncologists and geriatricians who treat cancer in the elderly.

4.2.3   Prognosis of Colorectal Cancer in Elderly Patients

Colorectal cancer provides a relatively prolonged survival: a survival rate of 79% at 1 year and 57% at 5 years. However, several studies have shown that age is an independent prognosis factor, as the survival rates of all cancers decrease with age (Vercelli et al. 2000). The Vercelli study that compared the survival rates of two groups of patients (aged 65 and over 65 years), at 1 year and 5 years, revealed a significant difference – regardless of the type of tumor – with a much lower survival rate at 1 year and 5 years in groups of older patients. The 1-year survival rate for men was 71% (aged 65–69), as opposed to 49% (aged 85 and over); the corresponding rates for women were 72% and 44%.

4.2.4   Under Inclusion of Elderly Patients in Clinical Trials

A literature review indicated a lack of data from clinical trials (Aapro et al. 2005). There is a clear underrepresentation of elderly patients in randomized trials of cancer (Hutchins et al. 1999). Hutchins et al. compared the percentage of patients over 65 included in the trials of the South West Oncology Group (SWOG) to that of the general population. Regardless of cancer site (with the exception of lymphomas), the percentage of patients over 65 was consistently below the proportion of people in the general population. The barriers to the inclusion of patients in the studies are numerous: the doctors' attitudes (most exclude patients based on age criteria alone), the eligibility criteria of the studies themselves that set an age limit or exclude some frequent comorbidities in the elderly, and the patients themselves and their families (Benson et al. 1991; Freyer et al. 1999; Townsley et al. 2003; Tyldesley et al. 2000). This lack of data from the literature prevents clinicians from basing optimal therapeutic management of elderly patients on research findings or recommendations (guidelines) (Fentiman et al. 1990). Groups of experts in geriatric oncology are currently working on developing recommendations for the management of colorectal cancer in the elderly (Aparicio et al. 2010).

4.2.5   Delay of Care for Elderly Patients

Whether at the screening, diagnosis, or treatment stage, there is suboptimal treatment of cancer in the elderly. Cancer is diagnosed at a more advanced stage than in younger subjects, thus worsening the prognosis (Diab et al. 2000; Tan et al. 2007). The delay of care is often multifactorial. Elderly patients usually consult several months after the onset of symptoms. Some symptoms, such as fatigue, weight loss, dyspnea, pain, constipation, and rectal bleeding, are often incorrectly attributed to advancing age. As a result, all diagnostic examinations are delayed. The presentation of the disease can be misleading (confusion, depression, impaired general condition, body pain). Further investigations are sometimes more difficult to perform in elderly patients (lack of preparation for colonoscopy, cardiovascular and respiratory complications related to anesthesia, colonic perforations) and often less frequent than in the young (Turner et al. 1999).

4.2.6   Suboptimal Treatment of Elderly Cancer Patients

Several studies have also shown that older patients are more at risk of inadequate treatment (over- or undertreatment) (Goodwin et al. 1993, 1996). Poor access to health care contributes to suboptimal treatment. Elderly patients are referred to a specialist practitioner less often because of their "potential vulnerability" that could complicate surgical management and/or oncology (Papamichael et al. 2009). A retrospective study of the French registry of digestive cancers showed that the treatment of stage III colorectal cancer varied according to age. In this study, treatment (surgery, adjuvant chemotherapy, radiotherapy) offered to patients over 75 did not include comorbidities, a clear indication of age discrimination in contrast to younger subjects (Quipourt et al. 2011). These results are confirmed by the study of Aparicio et al., where half (48%) the patients received suboptimal treatment of colorectal cancer that included metastatic tumors (Aparicio et al. 2009). Some factors related to surgical management directly influence the prognosis. The surgeries are more often done in an emergency context rather than a scheduled one (12% for patients over 80 vs. 5% for those under 65 in the case of rectal cancer; 17% for those over 80 years vs. 12%

for those under 65 in the case of colon cancer). Postoperative mortality is significantly higher in the elderly. In patients over 80, 6% of deaths occurred during hospitalization and 29% within 1 year of the intervention. In this study, predictors of poor outcome were the high number of comorbidities and the stage of cancer (Kunitake et al. 2010). Therefore, the later diagnosis of cancer in the elderly and inadequate cancer treatment in relation to the actual health status of the patient often render the management of cancer in the elderly suboptimal.

4.3   Special Features of the Care for Elderly Cancer Patients

4.3.1   Heterogeneity of the Cancer Population

One of the difficulties in managing elderly cancer patients is the heterogeneity of this population. All individuals do not age in the same way or at the same speed. Some patients suffer from multiple comorbidities; others have none. Some patients are completely dependent, while others retain complete autonomy, even in old age.

4.3.2   Impact of Comorbidities

The underlying health status of elderly patients interacts with the diagnostic and therapeutic decisions, thus preventing at times standard treatment. Age is not the only determinant. Several studies have shown the impact of comorbidities in the treatment of colon cancer. In the study by Janssen-Heijnen et al., the patients treated for colorectal cancer had surgery, regardless of their age and comorbidities (Janssen-Heijnen et al. 2007). Patients operated on in emergency; patients with comorbid conditions, such as cardiovascular, thromboembolic events, diabetes, and/or chronic bronchitis, had more postoperative complications and a higher mortality. In the case of colon surgery, patients over 80 suffered more pulmonary complications and a higher mortality (13%) than those under 80 (2%). In the case of rectal surgery, patients over 80 suffered significantly more bleeding complications, cardiovascular, renal failure, and death. In multivariate analysis, the risk of death increased with age and comorbidities. Assessing comorbidities and risk of decompensation is a major step in the management of elderly patients, with special attention being paid to the very elderly.

4.3.3   Specific Attention for Cognitive Impairment

Among all geriatric diseases, the special case of dementia is the most complex. In the study by Raji et al., the diagnosis of dementia was associated with a delayed diagnosis of cancer (including colorectal cancer) occurring at a later stage and with increased mortality from all causes (cancer-related or not). Survival also decreased when the diagnosis of dementia was made before the cancer (Raji et al. 2008). Dementia is a major cause of undertreatment in elderly cancer patients.

With the expansion of surgical indications in the elderly, one of the major post-operative complications is delirium. Because of previous unfortunate experiences involving a high prevalence of delirium during cancer treatments – whatever their intensity – health-care teams are reluctant to propose any cancer treatment whatsoever. Delirium and dementia are related: two-thirds of delirium syndromes occur in patients with dementia. Delirium has major implications in terms of loss of autonomy, morbidity, and mortality. A study of postoperative delirium was conducted among subjects over 75 who were to benefit from serious abdominal surgery. One-quarter of the operated patients presented postoperative delirium. The average length of stay was significantly higher for these patients (19 ± 11 days vs. 14 ± 8 days); postoperative mortality was significantly higher after delirium (14% vs. 9%). An ASA score greater than 3, impaired mobility (defined as a timed up and go test >20 s), and postoperative administration of tramadol were major risk factors for delirium, justifying a preoperative geriatric assessment (Brouquet et al. 2010).

Literature review shows that a history of cognitive impairment, advanced age, the preoperative use of psychotropic drugs, and a high number of comorbidities are also high-risk factors for postoperative delirium (Dasgupta and Dumbrell 2006). The prevalence of delirium also raises the issue of cost, due to the increase in length of stay, bedridden complications, decompensation of underlying diseases, risk of dependency, and workload (Sieber 2009). Postoperative delirium is a major problem in the surgical management of cancers, notably cancer of the colon. A delirium risk assessment must be offered to all patients to whom abdominal surgery is proposed, during the anesthesia and/or surgery consultation. Preventive measures can be proposed at that time (Inouye 2006; Inouye et al. 1999; Retornaz et al. 2010).

4.3.4   How to Assess the Underlying Conditions of Elderly Cancer Patients

In oncology, antineoplastic treatment is usually standardized: each type of cancer requires a particular combination of treatments, protocol, and order. In the case of colon cancer, treatment consists mainly of surgery, chemotherapy based on 5-fluorouracil, and targeted therapies. This relative standardization does not always apply to elderly patients. Comorbidities, disability, cognitive impairment, depression, mobility impairment, malnutrition, polypharmacy, and social context may interfere with the management of the cancer. Some nonspecific diseases can directly impact the treatment decision. For example, parameters such as malnutrition and renal failure may interfere directly with the pharmacokinetic of the chemotherapy and require an adaptation to reduce the risk of toxicities. The presence of severe neuropathy can indicate that a platinum-based chemotherapy should be avoided. The question of adjuvant chemotherapy is even more complex. Given after the tumor is removed to reduce the risk of recurrence or distant metastases, this chemotherapy can cause immediate toxicities that will aggravate the health of the patient without providing the potential benefit.

Table 4.1 Areas and main assessment tools used in standardized geriatric assessment in oncology

Areas assessed	Main tools
Functional status	ECOG-PS
	ADL (version Katz)
	IADL (version Lawton)
	IADL (version OARS à 14, 21, 29 items)
Comorbidities	CIRG-S, Charlson index, Satariano index
Drugs	Number, drug interactions
Cognition	MMSE, BOMC, clock-drawing test
Depression	GDS (4, 5, 15 items), HADS
Nutrition	BMI, MNA, weight loss
Mobility	TUG, Tinetti test, falls

ECOG PS Eastern Cooperative Oncology Group performance status, *ADL* basic activities of daily living, *IADL* instrumental activities of daily living, *CIRS-G* cumulative illness rating scale for geriatrics, *MMSE* Mini Mental Status Examination, *BOMC* Blessed Orientation-Memory-Concentration, *GDS* Geriatric Depression Scale, *HADS* Hospital Anxiety and Depression Scale, *BMI* body mass index, *MNA* Mini Nutritional Assessment, *TUG* Timed Up and Go test

4.3.5   Comprehensive Geriatric Assessment

The American National Comprehensive Cancer Network (NCCN) (Carreca et al. 2005) and the International Society of Geriatric Oncology (SIOG) (Extermann et al. 2005) both very involved in geriatric oncology research, and numerous literature reviews (Balducci and Beghe 2000; Bernabei et al. 2000; Chen et al. 2004; Misra et al. 2004; Repetto et al. 2003) propose the use of a comprehensive geriatric assessment (CGA) to determine optimal oncologic care, on the basis of the patient's health status rather than empirically. The CGA is a multidisciplinary evaluation in which potential problems of an older person are identified, listed, and explained, if possible; the economic and physical resources of the patient are identified; and a coordinated plan is proposed to target interventions in the issues identified in this patient (Solomon et al. 2003). Several randomized studies have shown that the CGA followed by interventions improves patients' functional status, prevents disability, reduces the risk of falls, reduces hospital readmissions and institutionalization, and reduces the incidence of mortality and costs (Cohen et al. 2002; Stuck et al. 1993). The main tools for CGA used in oncology are detailed in Table 4.1. The CGA is recommended for cancer patients so as to detect the vulnerability of these patients, estimate their tolerance to cancer treatment, define the optimal treatment, and determine the plans for those patients having multiple health problems related or unrelated to their underlying cancer.

4.3.6   Limitations of CGA

Several recent literature reviews, however, have questioned the real value of the CGA in geriatric oncology (Ferrucci et al. 2003; Maas et al. 2007). The limitations of the CGA are probably related to the target population. Indeed, the CGA was designed and validated for a population of older persons with disabilities and multiple diseases, who are hospitalized in geriatric wards, and/or require multiple interventions at home. It has not proven of interest in older adults without disabilities who live at home with a single medical condition, albeit it severe, i.e., in patients having relatively good underlying health (Ferrucci et al. 2003). According to the literature data, 70–80% of patients referred to oncology are independent for ADL (domestic activities of daily living), 50% are independent for IADL, half have no comorbidity, and 60% have a normal cognitive status. The older cancer patients represent a population that differs from the traditional geriatric patients: they have fewer comorbidities and good functional and underlying health status at the time of diagnosis. On the other hand, these patients have a higher prevalence of certain frailty markers such as malnutrition and impaired mobility. It is to be hoped that, in the future, a specific oncologic geriatric assessment "SOGA" will be developed, specifically tailored to older cancer patients, and adjustable according to the type of cancer and proposed treatment, with varying implications in terms of management.

4.3.7   When Should a CGA Be Proposed?

In oncology, many factors can interfere with the results of the CGA. Currently, patients are often sent to the geriatrician after surgery or after initiation of chemotherapy. These treatments, however, can affect the results of the CGA. The patient should ideally be evaluated right after the diagnosis of cancer and before any treatment.

It is also important to consider the impact of the cancer on the health of the patient at the time of CGA. For example, the classification of a patient suffering rapid weight loss, marked fatigue, and loss of autonomy related to aggressive or advanced cancer, as a "fragile subject," can conceivably change with optimal cancer treatment. The patient should, therefore, not be refused an aggressive cancer treatment. In the case of a patient who suffers progressive loss of weight and autonomy during the year preceding the cancer, the results of CGA will reflect the alteration of the reserves prior to the onset of the illness. This patient is considered vulnerable before the diagnosis of cancer, and there are risks of major toxicity, probably due to the underlying fragility (Fig. 4.1).

4.3.8   How to Identify Patients Who Need a CGA?

Currently, no recommendations from prospective randomized studies regarding the place of the CGA in cancer treatment are available, even though the various societies favor its use. Several teams are working on the validation of "screening" tools to identify patients requiring a CGA, for it cannot be offered to all patients, given the available resources and costs. In France, the objective of the "Oncodage" trial is to validate a questionnaire entitled "G8" that determines whether a CGA is necessary before the introduction of treatment, particularly chemotherapy. The G8 considers seven items of the MNA (Mini Nutritional Assessment), together with chronological age and perceived health status. The results should be available in 2012. Other teams

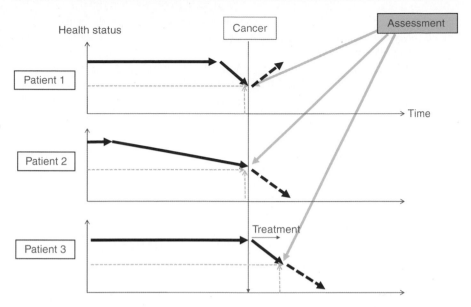

Fig. 4.1 Impact of cancer burden on the result of the assessment. *Explanation*: It is very important to consider the impact of the cancer on the health of the patient at the time of assessment. All three patients have similar health status at the time of assessment. Patient 1 suffers rapid weight loss, marked fatigue, and loss of mobility related to aggressive or advanced cancer. His classification as a "frail patient" can dramatically change with optimal cancer treatment. This patient should, therefore, not be refused an aggressive cancer treatment. Patient 2 suffers progressive loss of weight and mobility during the year preceding the cancer. The results of assessment will reflect the alteration of the reserves prior to the onset of the cancer. This patient is considered vulnerable before the diagnosis of cancer, and there are risks of major toxicities with aggressive therapies. For Patient 3, the assessment is done only after the start of cancer treatment. The result of your assessment may reflect the impact of the treatment rather than the underlying patient heath status. Continuing these treatment will probably lead to toxicities

use the VES-13 as a screening tool or the a-CGA, although both have not been validated in various cancer types and in many patients (Luciani et al. 2010; Overcash et al. 2010). The use of frailty markers as a tool for screening patients (Retornaz et al. 2008) or as a predictor of toxicity is potentially a new way of research in oncologic (Puts et al. 2011) or surgery settings (Makary et al. 2010; Tan et al. 2011).

4.4   Specific Issues Concerning Chemotherapy in Elderly Patients

4.4.1   Can the Patient Tolerate Chemotherapy?

Choosing the optimal treatment regimen for an elderly patient, in terms of schema and dose, is challenging because one must take into account not only the physiological changes associated with aging but also the pathological changes which are added over time. The various types of chemotherapy do not all have the same toxicity profile. Myelosuppression is the main toxic effect of most chemotherapy agents, predisposing the patient for infections. Fever requires prompt treatment. The administration of leukocyte growth factors can limit the effects of myelosuppression; these agents are recommended by the SIOG in chemotherapy having high myelosuppressive effects. Nausea and vomiting are not more frequent in elderly patients, but their consequences are more severe (dehydration, malnutrition). On the other hand, elderly patients are at increased risk of gastrointestinal toxicity, such as mucosal damage (mucositis) and diarrhea, due to a decrease in the turnover time of the digestive epithelium. If possible, these side effects should be prevented (mouthwashes, antidiarrheals) and actively treated (intravenous or subcutaneous infusion). Other toxicities such as neurotoxicity are often overlooked in oncology, even though they have a major impact on elderly patients. Some drugs (e.g., platinum salts) lead to neuropathies responsible for disabling pain, gait disturbance leading to increased risk of falling, loss of autonomy, etc. The fatigue caused by chemotherapy can also cause a loss of autonomy. Even without training in oncology, the geriatrician should ideally know, when assessing the patient, the proposed chemotherapy regimen and potential toxicities or the assistance of the oncologist as to the potential toxicity of the proposed processing.

Most types of chemotherapy are administered with drugs that limit the side effects of the treatment. However, these drugs have their own side effects that can be just as deleterious in the elderly. For instance, antiemetic drugs may lead to constipation that must be prevented. Steroids are also often administered as a bolus before the infusion of chemotherapy and are a source of glycemic decompensation or delirium. Again, a good knowledge of the entire proposed treatment is the key to preventing side effects.

Adjuvant chemotherapy requires special attention when a patient is assessed by a geriatrician. In fact, this chemotherapy is delivered after curative treatment (usually surgery) to reduce the risk of recurrence or metastasis by destroying islet cell cancer that could escape from the tumor before surgery and nest in different organs. The chemotherapy can, however, cause toxicities that can aggravate the condition of the patient without providing the potential benefit. Statistically speaking, patients are more likely to survive with adjuvant chemotherapy than without, but, for any given patient, the complications of chemotherapy can destroy the expected positive effects. Administering chemotherapy (of which the expected theoretical benefit is the reduction of the risk of recurrence or metastases within 5 years) to vulnerable patients exposes them to a high risk of complications and a risk of early death; any benefit from the treatment is lost (e.g., decompensation cascade evolving from a loss of autonomy). The geriatrician should try to determine whether the overall life expectancy of the patient is greater than the risk of relapse and whether any underlying factors may increase the risk of toxicity. To calculate the overall life expectancy, the geriatrician can use predictive tools of mortality such as the Walter score (score at 1 year) or the Lee score (score at 4 years) (Lee et al. 2006; Walter et al. 2001).

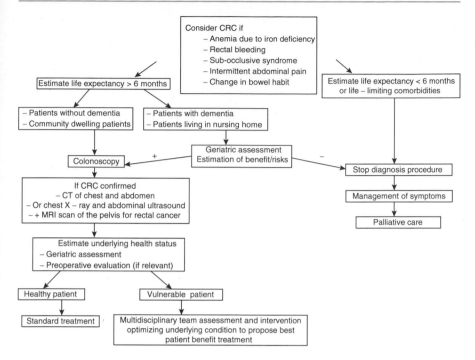

Fig. 4.2 Decision making algorithm from diagnosis to treatment decision. *CRC* Colorectal cancer

Two recent studies have provided predictive tools for toxicity from chemotherapy in the elderly (Extermann et al. 2011; Hurria et al. 2011). However, these are too complex for everyday use.

Conclusion

Till today, older colorectal cancer patients have delayed diagnosis and receive suboptimal treatment. Elderly patients should be exposed to more aggressive management more similar to their counterparts.

Due to the heterogeneity of the elderly patient population, patients over 65 years of age need to undergo preoperative evaluation, which should include a cancer-specific assessment as well as a whole patient evaluation for the most common physiological effects of aging, physical and mental ability, and social support (Fig. 4.2). A geriatric team should be involved in patient management in the case of a patient with comorbidities or poor health status.

Age alone should not be a barrier to treatment. Patients should receive the most intensive and appropriate treatment thought to be safe and effective according to their underlying health status and comorbidities.

References

Aapro MS, Kohne CH, Cohen HJ et al (2005) Never too old? Age should not be a barrier to enrolment in cancer clinical trials. Oncologist 10:198–204

Aouba A, Péquignot F, Le Toullec A, et al (2007) Les causes médicales de décès en France en 2004 et leur évolution 1980–2004. Bulletin Epidémiologique Hebdomadaire 35–36:308–14. http://www.insee.fr

Aparicio T, Mitry E, Sa Cunha A et al (2005) Management of colorectal cancer of elderly patients. Gastroenterol Clin Biol 29:1014–1023

Aparicio T, Navazesh A, Boutron I et al (2009) Half of elderly patients routinely treated for colorectal cancer receive a sub-standard treatment. Crit Rev Oncol Hematol 71:249–257

Aparicio T, Bouché O, Carola E et al (2010) Recommandations du GEPOG (Groupe d' Echanges et de Pratique en Onco-Geriatrie) pour le traitement des cancers colorectaux métastatiques des patients âgés. Journal d'Onco-Gériatrie 3(4):157–163

Balducci L, Beghe C (2000) The application of the principles of geriatrics to the management of the older person with cancer. Crit Rev Oncol Hematol 35:147–154

Benson AB III, Pregler JP, Bean JA et al (1991) Oncologists' reluctance to accrue patients onto clinical trials: an Illinois Cancer Center study. J Clin Oncol 9:2067–2075

Bernabei R, Venturiero V, Tarsitani P et al (2000) The comprehensive geriatric assessment: when, where, how. Crit Rev Oncol Hematol 33:45–56

Brouquet A, Cudennec T, Benoist S et al (2010) Impaired mobility, ASA status and administration of tramadol are risk factors for postoperative delirium in patients aged 75 years or more after major abdominal surgery. Ann Surg 251:759–765

Carreca I, Balducci L, Extermann M (2005) Cancer in the older person. Cancer Treat Rev 31:380–402

Chen CC, Kenefick AL, Tang ST et al (2004) Utilization of comprehensive geriatric assessment in cancer patients. Crit Rev Oncol Hematol 49:53–67

Dasgupta M, Dumbrell AC (2006) Preoperative risk assessment for delirium after noncardiac surgery: a systematic review. J Am Geriatr Soc 54:1578–1589

Diab SG, Elledge RM, Clark GM (2000) Tumor characteristics and clinical outcome of elderly women with breast cancer. J Natl Cancer Inst 92:550–556

Extermann M, Aapro M, Bernabei R, Task Force on CGA of the International Society of Geriatric Oncology et al (2005) Use of comprehensive geriatric assessment in older cancer patients: recommendations from the task force on CGA of the International Society of Geriatric Oncology (SIOG). Crit Rev Oncol Hematol 55:241–252

Extermann M, Boler I, Reich RR et al (2011) Predicting the risk of chemotherapy toxicity in older patients: the Chemotherapy Risk Assessment Scale for High-Age Patients (CRASH) score. Cancer. doi:10.1002/cncr.26646

Fentiman IS, Tirelli U, Monfardini S et al (1990) Cancer in the elderly: why so badly treated? Lancet 335:1020–1022

Ferrucci L, Guralnik JM, Cavazzini C et al (2003) The frailty syndrome: a critical issue in geriatric oncology. Crit Rev Oncol Hematol 46:127–137

Goodwin JS, Hunt WC, Samet JM (1993) Determinants of cancer therapy in elderly patients. Cancer 72:594–601

Goodwin JS, Samet JM, Hunt WC (1996) Determinants of survival in older cancer patients. J Natl Cancer Inst 88:1031–38. http://www.iinsee.fr

Hurria A, Togawa K, Mohile SG et al (2011) Predicting chemotherapy toxicity in older adults with cancer: a prospective multicenter study. J Clin Oncol 29:3457–3465

Hutchins LF, Unger JM, Crowley JJ et al (1999) Underrepresentation of patients 65 years of age or older in cancer-treatment trials. N Engl J Med 341:2061–2067

Inouye S (2006) Delirium in older persons. N Engl J Med 354:1157–1165

Inouye S, Bogardus S, Charpentier P et al (1999) A multicomponent intervention to prevent delirium in hospitalized older patients. N Engl J Med 340:669–676

Janssen-Heijnen ML, Maas HA, Houterman S et al (2007) Comorbidity in older surgical cancer patients: influence on patient care and outcome. Eur J Cancer 43(15):2179–2193

Kunitake H, Zingmond D, Ryoo J et al (2010) Caring for octogenarian and nonagenarian patients with colorectal cancer: what should our standards and expectations be? Dis Colon Rectum 53:735–743

Lee SJ, Lindquist K, Segal MR et al (2006) Development and validation of a prognostic index for 4-year mortality in older adults. JAMA 295:801–808

Luciani A, Ascione G, Bertuzzi C et al (2010) Detecting disabilities in older patients with cancer: comparison between comprehensive geriatric assessment and vulnerable elders survey-13. J Clin Oncol 28:2046–2050

Maas HA, Janssen-Heijnen ML, Olde Rikkert MG et al (2007) Comprehensive geriatric assessment and its clinical impact in oncology. Eur J Cancer 43:2161–2169

Makary MA, Segev DL, Pronovost PJ et al (2010) Frailty as a predictor of surgical outcomes in older patients. J Am Coll Surg 210:901–908

Misra D, Seo PH, Cohen HJ (2004) Aging and cancer. Clin Adv Hematol Oncol 2:457–465

Papamichael D, Audisio R, Horiot J-C et al (2009) Treatment of the elderly colorectal cancer patient: SIOG expert recommendations. Ann Oncol 16:20–25

Puts MT, Monette J, Girre V et al (2011) Are frailty markers useful for predicting treatment toxicity and mortality in older newly diagnosed cancer patients? Results from a prospective pilot study. Crit Rev Oncol Hematol 78:138–149

Quipourt V, Jooste V, Cottet V et al (2011) Comorbidities alone do not explain the undertreatment of colorectal cancer in older adults: a French population-based study. J Am Geriatr Soc 59:694–698

Raji M, Kuo Y-F, Freeman J et al (2008) Effect of a dementia diagnosis on survival of older patients after a diagnosis of breast, colon, or prostate cancer implications for cancer care. Arch Intern Med 168:2033–2040

Repetto L, Venturino A, Fratino L et al (2003) Geriatric oncology: a clinical approach to the older patient with cancer. Eur J Cancer 39:870–880

Retornaz F, Monette J, Batist G et al (2008) Usefulness of frailty markers in the assessment of health and functional status of older cancer patients referred for chemotherapy: a pilot study. J Gerontol A Biol Sci Med Sci 63:518–522

Retornaz F, Potard I, Molines C et al (2010) Quand l'équipe gériatrique restaure la confiance de l'équipe médico-chirurgicale. Journal d'Onco-Gériatrie 1:33–36

Sieber F (2009) Post operative delirium in the elderly surgical patient. Anesthesiol Clin 27:451–464

Stuck AE, Siu AL, Wieland GD et al (1993) Comprehensive geriatric assessment: a meta-analysis of controlled trials. Lancet 342:1032–1036

Tan E, Tilney H, Thompson M et al (2007) The United Kingdom national bowel cancer project – epidemiology and surgical risk in the elderly. Eur J Cancer 43:2285–2294

Tan KY, Kawamura YJ, Tokomitsu A et al (2011) Assessment for frailty is useful for predicting morbidity in elderly patients undergoing colorectal cancer resection whose comorbidities are already optimized. Am J Surg [Epub ahead of print]

Turner N, Haward R, Mulley G et al (1999) Cancer in old age: is it inadequately investigated and treated? BMJ 319:309–312

Townsley CA, Naidoo K, Pond GR et al (2003) Are older cancer patients being referred to oncologists? A mail questionnaire of Ontario primary care practitioners to evaluate their referral patterns. J Clin Oncol 21:4627–4635

Tyldesley S, Zhang-Salomons J, Groome PA et al (2000) Association between age and the utilization of radiotherapy in Ontario. Int J Radiat Oncol Biol Phys 47:469–480

Vercelli M, Capocaccia R, Quaglia A et al (2000) Relative survival in elderly European cancer patients: evidence for health care inequalities. The EUROCARE Working Group. Crit Rev Oncol Hematol 35:161–179

Walter LC, Brand RJ, Counsell SR et al (2001) Development and validation of a prognostic index for 1-year mortality in older adults after hospitalization. JAMA 285(23):2987–2994

Yancik R, Ries LA (2000) Aging and cancer in America. Demographic and epidemiologic perspectives. Hematol Oncol Clin North Am 14:17–23

Surgical Considerations Prior to Colorectal Cancer Surgery

5

Isaac Seow-En and Francis Seow-Choen

Take Home Pearls

- Age is not the sole criterion against the use of surgery for colorectal cancer.
- The elderly should be optimized for surgery and surgery carried out as soon as practicable.
- The aims of treatment should be well spelt out to ensure a satisfactory outcome from all sides.
- Appropriate informed consent and understanding of the elderly and their families are important before surgery.

5.1   Introduction

The Chinese have a saying: 'the family with an aged person has a precious treasure'. Age in itself is not a problem. However with age comes deterioration of somatic and psychosocial functions, health and a less favourable response to trauma including surgical stress (Tan et al. 2010). As we assess the elderly coming with various medical conditions for surgical correction, we have to consider the elderly as a whole person within the environment of their daily life. There are other chapters in this book that deal with psychosocial, nursing, rehabilitative management of co-morbid conditions,

I. Seow-En, MBBS
Resident, Seow-Choen Colorectal Surgery PLC,
290 Orchard Road Paragon #06-06,
Singapore 238859, Singapore

F. Seow-Choen, MBBS, FAMS, FRCSEd (✉)
Medical Director, Fortis Colorectal Hospital,
19 Adam Road, Singapore 289891, Singapore
e-mail: seowchoen@colorectalcentre.com

K.-Y. Tan (ed.), *Colorectal Cancer in the Elderly*,   47
DOI 10.1007/978-3-642-29883-7_5, © Springer-Verlag Berlin Heidelberg 2013

assessment of fitness for surgery, etc. Therefore in this chapter, we will confine our-
selves to what we consider surgical considerations prior to surgery for the elderly.
In this regard, colorectal surgeons have to be especially careful as a great majority of
their patients are 'elderly'. We have avoided in this chapter any designation or definition
of the word elderly with regard to chronological age. As health providers, we are all
well aware that chronological age does not correlate exactly with biological age. We
have treated and even operated on nonagenarians who have been healthier than sexa-
genarians with regard to physical and psychological body functions. So as we discuss
surgical considerations in the elderly, we talk of those who are not just elderly in
chronological age but also of those who might not be so old in chronological age but
whose somatic conditions qualify them as elderly. Age alone therefore is not a predictor
of major complications after colorectal surgery including laparoscopic surgery. Elderly
people with colorectal cancers or its complications should not be denied elective surgery (Tan et al. 2006). An elderly person with no co-morbidities will do better than a
younger person with multiple co-morbidities. Furthermore, it had been noted before
that it is not the individual co-morbidity but the quantification of overall co-morbidities that are important in predicting perioperative mortality (Tan et al. 2011).

5.2   Assessment for Surgery in the Elderly

The surgical management of the elderly often revolves not just on the surgery itself
but also on the co-management of a whole host of other co-morbid conditions which
may make the patient at high risk for anaesthesia and surgery. This subject is discussed in another chapter but suffice to say here that adequate pre-surgical preparation and the involvement of other specialists may be vital to good outcome in such
patients. Conditions which are reversible must be carefully looked at and corrected;
including but not limited to fluid and electrolyte abnormalities and other co-morbid
conditions. However, it must also be said that many such conditions may be optimized but they may not necessarily be totally reversible. Such is the effect of age on
the human frame. In such situations, it behoves the surgeon to recognize the situation as such and get on with the patient who is the fittest he will ever be without the
needed surgery. Early surgery in such patients will be life saving (Lan et al. 2000).
Surgery for colorectal cancer should be performed early once the patient is optimized. A short period of prehabilitation may improve surgical outcomes. However,
postponement of surgical intervention until tumour complications arise is more
likely to be associated with a poorer outcome (Tan et al. 2006).

5.3   Tailoring the Indications for Surgery
         to the Needs of the Elderly

The time will come, after all co-morbid imbalances and problems have been corrected and the patient now declared as fit as he will ever be, for the timing and
approach to surgery to be discussed with the patient. Indications for colorectal cancer surgery are often considered under two subdivisions: (1) surgical conditions

Table 5.1 Common indications for surgery in the elderly with colorectal cancer

1. Curative resection of primary/recurrent colorectal cancer
2. Palliative resection of primary/recurrent colorectal cancer
3. Resection of cancer for bleeding/anaemia
4. Resection/diversional procedures for intestinal obstruction
5. Restoration of intestinal continuity/closure of stomas
6. Management of cancer-related intestinal fistula
7. Resection of secondary cancers,
   e.g. Krukenberg's tumours, Sister Joseph's nodule, etc.
8. Surgical procedures for relief of biliary obstruction
9. Surgical procedures for relief of ureteric obstruction
10. Surgical procedures for relief of ascites/pleural effusion

where surgery is mandatory and (2) surgical conditions where surgery is one of the options. In truth, these are false divisions. A sensible approach to the management of these elderly patients is of utmost importance in obtaining a good outcome. The treatment goals need not necessarily be the same as those of surgical treatment for someone much younger or fitter.

The timing and type of surgery undertaken must be carefully thought out. The surgeon managing an elderly person should have at his disposal good knowledge of all the possible techniques of dealing with the particular problem faced by the elderly under his care. Not all the commonly encountered problems seen in the elderly patient must be dealt with by surgery alone (Table 5.1).

The most efficacious treatment of curative colorectal cancer is still surgical extirpation. Where the patient is fit, surgery still remains the simplest and easiest method of curing a patient presenting with colorectal cancer. For potentially curable colorectal cancer, no effort should be spared to ensure and optimize patients for surgery. This statement however should be moderated in patients where the frailty of age or the presence of severe disease demands. It is still a truth that a live patient with a potentially deadly cancer is still better than a dead patient with all cancer in his body removed. Having said this however, the surgeon should not shrug off the responsibility of a thorough explanation and discussion of the purpose of surgery or any other treatment with the patient and relatives. The risks and benefits of each technique or procedure should be carefully weighed, assessed and tailored to the preference of the patient. The patient's goal for accepting treatment must be elucidated. If the patient and family accept the risks and benefits of surgery, the surgeon should then be prepared to go ahead and perform the surgery as skilfully as possible.

5.3.1   Examples of Surgical Decision Making in the Elderly

We recently treated an elderly 91-year-old lady who was relatively fit. She had just recovered from pneumonia and her infection had cleared. Her only other co-morbid factor was early dementia but otherwise she was communicative and had a positive outlook. Her relatives explained that she had good long-term memory retention but that she had very poor short-term memory. She had been seen by another surgeon who had diagnosed cancer at 9 cm from the anal verge and advised her for abdominal perineal resection. CT scan revealed the cancer to be T2N0M0 stage. After speaking with the original surgeon, it was found that the reason for advising an abdominal perineal resection was the age of the patient and location of the cancer. Her relatives were frightened at the prospect of managing a stoma bag, and the patient herself was unable to grasp the concept of a stoma. We had a thorough discussion regarding life expectancy for a 91-year-old and the sort of surgery that would be least intrusive and traumatic as well as the possibilities of needing any sort of stoma bag including the use of a defunctioning stoma. It was elucidated that the patient felt that having a stoma would greatly reduce her quality of life. It was decided that her goal was to continue to have good quality life, and she was not too particular about her life expectancy. We thus planned for a laparoscopic low anterior resection without a total mesorectal excision, accepting a higher risk of inadequate oncological clearance. However in doing so, we were able to perform primary anastomosis without the need for a defunctioning stoma and her post-operative bowel function would be better. And indeed she recovered well and was discharged 3 days following surgery.

In the palliative setting, the same considerations prevail. If surgery is the best way to moderate the effects of the disease, then the good surgeon should thoroughly explain this to the patient and relatives and do whatever is needed for the patient to have a life that is meaningful. Where surgery is not needed, then the alternatives should be carefully explained and the patient advised accordingly. We recently saw an elderly patient with a sigmoid cancer which was not obstructing and was in fact asymptomatic. He was being investigated as routine blood tests showed an extremely high carcinoembryonic antigen level. PET scan showed massive liver replacement by secondaries and there were lung metastases as well. He was referred for chemotherapy but 3 months into this therapy, he developed abdominal distension and evidence of intestinal obstruction at the sigmoid cancer level. Further imaging revealed minimal response to the chemotherapy. Major surgery including laparoscopic surgery may indeed improve his symptoms, but it also had the risk of causing detrimental effect on his life expectancy and short-term quality of life. We decided therefore to advise him for an intraluminal colonic metal stent. This was inserted with a good response and the patient was asymptomatic thereafter for a further 6 months before he died from advanced disease.

In situations where the effects of the disease are such that treatment is urgently needed but where the co-morbid state of the patient contradicts extirpative surgery, other less risky alternatives should be sought and discussed with the patient and caregivers. An example of this was a patient we saw with advanced recurrent colorectal cancer with metastases to the peritoneum, liver and lung. He presented to us during palliative chemotherapy with recurrent intestinal obstruction. The patient was in obvious pain and distress, and the abdomen was severely distended with a midline scar and a left iliac fossa end colostomy. Blood investigations revealed severe hypoproteinaemia and CT scan showed small bowel obstruction by likely peritoneal nodules. It would have been easy for us to dismiss this problem as being untreatable and to advise continuous nasogastric suction and increase in the prescription of pain killers. However, together with the patient, we decided that we should make life more meaningful for this patient if we could enable him to eat and defaecate and would thereby also decrease his pain. We performed a water-soluble contrast follow through to get a better picture of the problem. Fortunately for the patient, we found the obstruction to be at the mid- to distal ileum. It was then reasonable to consider performing a small procedure to divert the bowel proximal to the obstruction. We planned for an ileostomy and decompression through a small right iliac fossa incision. If that had failed, we had counselled the patient that then purely palliative measures would be appropriate. As it went, we managed to do a hassle-free procedure and the patient recovered quickly and was able to eat and defaecate for about 7 months before succumbing to massive liver secondaries.

5.4   Practical Aspects on Consent for Surgery in the Elderly

Most elderly patients are able to make decisions regarding surgery and other options for treatment on their own (Table 5.2). Some however are dependent on their relatives to make these decisions for them. This sort of situations are not infrequently encountered and may be due to deteriorating mental function of these elderly, lack of understanding of the elderly regarding the intricacies of the proposed treatment, dependence on relatives for housing or other financial support or even just due to relatives who want to take control over these elderly relatives. These issues vary depending on the patient's racial and cultural background. Obtaining consent for treatment and surgery in the elderly is therefore often a difficult process. Where the elderly patients are able to understand and want to take the responsibility themselves, this process may be quicker but the surgeon will often find younger members of the family or extended family who will then raise other issues or problems and insists on another round of explanation. Sometimes in patients with large families, these sorts of family meetings can be repeated with different relatives claiming to be the one in the need to know and the one to make the ultimate decision on treatment.

Our advice is to make sure that the patient is at the centre of all these discussions. It is important to make every effort for the elderly patient to understand his or her medical condition and the rationale of the suggested treatment and alternative options. A unified goal of treatment needs to be determined between the surgical team and the patient. For an elderly patient with chronic illnesses and disabilities, long-term survival may not be the most important priority; loss of independence,

Table 5.2 Information to be given to patients when obtaining consent

1. The reason and purpose of the intended surgery in the language understood by the patient and relatives
2. Other options available or not suitable for the particular patient and his condition
3. The likely risk and benefits of the surgical procedure
4. The operating surgeon should be the one taking consent, but if he is not the one, an explanation of who will be in charge should be given
5. A reminder to the patient that he or she has the right to another opinion and that he or she can refuse consent at any time even after signing

quality of life and burden on caregivers may take precedence. It has been shown that the preference of the patient may differ widely from what the surrogate and physicians' understanding of their preference may be (Tan et al. 2010). As such, a thorough understanding of the patient's preferences and priorities is important in this decision-making process, and good patient education facilitates elucidating of these preferences when the patient understands more about their condition and potential best and worst outcomes.

Where the patient is of sound mind and able to comprehend all the intricacies of treatment, the patient should be the one to make the final decision regarding treatment. In all situations but especially in a multicultural or multi-language environment, it is imperative that the surgeon speaks simply and clearly with the patient and his relatives to avoid any misunderstanding. It is imperative, for the patient's and surgeon's sake, that explanations regarding surgery involve as many members of the immediate family as possible. Family dynamics are often not clear and many families have many other reasons why an elderly should or should not have the recommended treatment, and many of these may or may not be medically based. In Asia, we often encounter the situation whereby members of the family for whatever reason good or bad press the surgeon to hide material facts regarding diagnosis or treatment from the patient himself. Sometimes their requests may be innocuous. Relatives may say that they do not want the patient to worry excessively and that the surgeon should not use the word cancer in discussing treatment but say something like tumour or growth instead. At other times, their requests may be downright misleading or untruthful. Our policy is to ask the patient whether they want to know of their condition; most elderly actually prefer to know the diagnosis than to be kept in the dark. All communications and issues discussed should be clearly documented for future reference.

Where the elderly patient is not capable of making the decision himself, a family conference should be called. The one responsible for all the decision making regarding the patient should be identified as early in this process as possible. The surgeon should satisfy himself by direct questioning of the relatives that this particular person is the one to make the final decision and is the contact person in all medical emergencies.

In many countries, patients may have to pay out of pocket for any surgical intervention. In such situations, the caregiver or the patient himself will have to undergo financial counselling and a detailed estimation of the entire cost of the surgery spelled out. The costs of each sort of surgery will vary from country to country and even within each country depending on whether payment is by insurance or government or by the patients themselves. The goals of treatment as well as the costs of achieving these goals must be discussed to avoid the situation where the patient may end up cured or worse still in worse health but without further financial capability to see himself through the future. In our practice, elderly patients with colorectal cancer are always told about the costs of laparoscopic surgery versus those of open surgery. The risks and benefits are thoroughly discussed to enable patients to make an informed decision about the effects of surgery on them but also about the effect of any financial burden on their resources following surgery.

5.5   Details of Surgical Procedure and Consent

There are three options possible as far as the amount and content of information to be given to patients prior to any medical intervention (Wheeler 2006). The first option is that of the exhaustive informed consent. Although laudable, this option is not practicable although the phraseology is thrown about often enough. The second option is that of what a group of reasonable surgeons would do in similar circumstances. This is by far the most commonly used principle and is known as the Bolam principle (Wheeler 2006). The third option is what a reasonable patient would want to know under the circumstances. This is again very reasonable place to start giving information.

What the surgeon should discuss during consent taking should be what any reasonable person would want to know before decisions can be made. By considering the position of the reasonable person, the surgeon would have fulfilled the legal requirements in obtaining consent. However, there is increasing scrutiny of the particular patients' particular circumstances. In recent years, there is an increasing dichotomy of views regarding what or who may be defined as being reasonable. Barriers to this process include reasons ranging from a lack of education, low intellectual quotient, deteriorating mental faculties, cultural barriers, social-psychological difficulties as well as many other reasons peculiar to the patient and family.

The Bolam principle established the criterion that reasonableness can be extrapolated by reference to the views of a group of comparable doctors. What is reasonable therefore from this point of view is what a group of doctors in the same situation with the same training would do.

Personally, we take the view that in our obtaining consent, we behave as a group of reasonable surgeons would and give the information they would consider relevant to the surgery at hand. We would at the same time also consider the point of view of the reasonable patient and expect that level of information to be given which would allow a non-surgically trained person to understand and digest the information sufficiently to make a good personal decision regarding what he or she ought to do in their situation. The current and prevailing view regarding consent for surgery is that surgeons have a personal duty to inform patients of the risks and benefits of the intended surgery in so far as those risks and benefits are commonly or specifically associated with the surgery in question. A practical approach is to provide information in these two following areas:
1. Common risks of the treatment and procedure
2. Less common risks but may have significant impact if they do occur

5.6   Patient Education

The undertaking of major surgery is a major life event for anyone, especially in the elderly patient where there are profound implications of increased dependence and risk of morbidity and mortality. This may not be recognized by the surgeon who

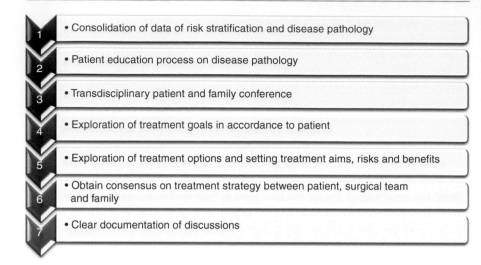

1 • Consolidation of data of risk stratification and disease pathology

2 • Patient education process on disease pathology

3 • Transdisciplinary patient and family conference

4 • Exploration of treatment goals in accordance to patient

5 • Exploration of treatment options and setting treatment aims, risks and benefits

6 • Obtain consensus on treatment strategy between patient, surgical team and family

7 • Clear documentation of discussions

Fig. 5.1 Alexandra Health, Khoo Teck Puat Hospital Geriatric Surgery Service step-wise consenting process

performs similar operations in frequently. Many patients, do not know what to expect and they have to deal with fears of the unknown. Patient and family education play an important role in alleviating these fears and have a positive impact on the patients' psyche for the operation.

The Alexandra Health Geriatric Surgery Service has a preoperative education package as part of the transdisciplinary approach to preoperative patient management. The nurse clinician takes on the role of the educator after the surgeon has discussed aspects of the surgery with the patient and family. The nurse clinician reinforces what the surgeon has said and furthermore educates the patient and family on what to expect in the perioperative period and what the patient has to do for himself/herself to ensure a good outcome. Examples of patients with similar conditions and operations can be shown to the patient and family to reassure patients of the high possibility of good surgical outcome. Patients are then likely to have a more positive outlook on their surgery. Compliance to treatment strategies may thus be improved.

This education process is part of the stepwise consenting process that is practiced by the service (Fig. 5.1).

Conclusion

Age by itself is not a risk factor in surgery for colorectal cancer in the elderly. Co-morbidities should be optimized and any surgery proposed should be done as soon as practical to prevent further complications from arising. Treatment goals must be well defined and the patient and their families should be well informed of what these treatment goals are as well as of the risks and benefits of the intended surgery.

References

Lan Q, Ikeda H, Jimbo H, Izumiyama H, Matsumoto K (2000) Considerations on surgical treatment for elderly patients with intracranial aneurysms. Surg Neurol 53:231–238

Tan KY, Chen CM, Ng C, Tan SM, Tay KH (2006) Which octogenarians do poorly after major open abdominal surgery in our Asian population. World J Surg 30:547–52

Tan KY, Kawamura Y, Mizokami K, Sasaki J, Tsujinaka S, Maeda T, Konishi F (2009) Colorectal surgery in octogenarian patients-outcomes and predictors of morbidity. Int J Colorectal Dis 24:185–189

Tan KY, Konishi F, Tan L, Chin WK, Ong HY, Tan P (2010) Optimizing the management of elderly colorectal surgery patients. Surg Today 40:999–1010

Tan KY, Konishi F, Kawamura Y, Maeda T, Sasaki J, Tsujinaka S, Horie H (2011) Laparoscopic colorectal surgery in elderly patients: a case–control study of 15 years of experience. Am J Surg 201:531–536

Wheeler R (2006) Consent in surgery. Ann R Coll Surg Engl 88:261–264

Psychosocial Considerations Prior to Surgery

6

Mary Rockwood Lane, Michael Samuels, and Emi Lenes

Take Home Pearls

- Enabling, sustaining, and honoring hope are important components before surgery.
- Human dignity of the patient is the upmost importance.
- Spirituality can be expressed in a diversity of ways.
- The utilization of art interventions can be a meaningful coping strategy.
- Guided imagery can be a powerful psychosocial preparation for surgery.
- Humor can potentially bring joy or offense to the presurgical experience.
- Jean Watson's caring science is based on the ethic of love.

> We are the light in institutional darkness, so I invite you to join me and return to the light of our humanity.
> – Jean Watson

M.R. Lane, PhD, RN, FAAN (✉)
University of Florida College of Nursing,
Gainesville, FL, USA
e-mail: maryrockwoodlane@gmail.com

M. Samuels, M.D.
John F. Kennedy University, College of Holistic Health,
Pleasant Hill, San Fransisco, USA

E. Lenes, EdS, NCC, LMHC
University of Florida College of Education,
Gainesville, FL, USA

K.-Y. Tan (ed.), *Colorectal Cancer in the Elderly*,
DOI 10.1007/978-3-642-29883-7_6, © Springer-Verlag Berlin Heidelberg 2013

6.1   Introduction

Jean Watson's theory of caring science is based on the ethic of love, which is necessary for healing and preparation for surgery. This moral, theoretical, and philosophical
foundation leads to an authentic caring relationship with each patient. Creative interventions will be presented in this chapter that can provide support and help prepare the
patients and caregivers for surgery. Preserving the diversity of each individuals experience promotes human dignity. Interdisciplinary collaboration and communication
places the patient and the patient's support system first. This promotes knowledge,
growth, and empowerment in which the patient enhances their faith in their own inner
resources to cope with the surgical experience.

6.1.1   Benefits of Psychosocial Preparation

Several benefits are possible from taking an active role in preparing for surgery. These
include:
- Less distress and anxiety both before and after surgery
- Less pain
- Faster return to health
- Shorter recovery period
- Reduced health-care demands due to empowering the patient to take more respon-
  sibility for their recovery
- Increased patient satisfaction and outcome

6.1.2   Some Causes of the Physical and Emotional
           Preoperative Surgical Stress

Understandably, surgery may cause people to have thoughts and fears about the
"unknown." Although upcoming surgery can cause uneasiness and discomfort,
patients can relax and even experience personal growth throughout a health crisis.
Some causes of stress include:
- Physical pain
- Feeling vulnerable and unconscious on the surgical table
- Fears of complications
- Fears about the recovery process
- Discomfort about keeping a colostomy bag clean and changed, if needed
  When a patient is responding to stress, the body can display some of the following
symptoms:
- Rapid and shallow breathing
- Increased muscle tension
- Release of stress hormones, like cortisol
- Increased heart rate and blood pressure
- Lowered immune system function
  Managing stress and pain as effectively as possible can influence one's recovery
in a positive way. The following ten Caritas Practices discuss ways health-care

professionals, patients, and family members can help alleviate some of the negative psychosocial repercussions.

6.1.3   How to Psychologically Prepare Patients for Surgery

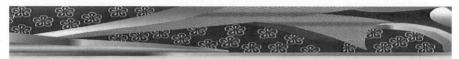

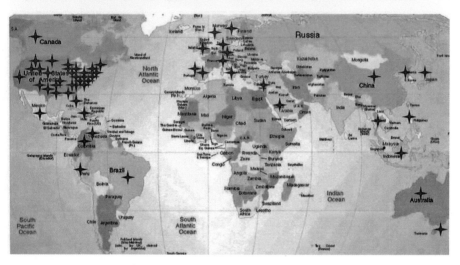

Adopting Watson's Caring Theory/Model: Joining a Global Movement
✦ Where Caring Theory/Model Has Been Adopted into Practice

6.2   Ten Caritas Processes

6.2.1   Caritas Process #1

Practicing Loving-Kindness and Equanimity Within the Context of Caring Consciousness

> Love is what we all are; we can lose the awareness of love, but not the state itself. That is not
> an option. Love is immovable.
> – Katie Bowan

Embracing altruistic values and practicing loving-kindness with self and others changes the patient's experience of surgery. When a caregiver looks at a patient with loving-kindness, a transpersonal relationship is started which can facilitate healing and successful outcomes. As Jean Watson (2008) stated so elegantly, finding loving-kindness within requires an inner pause to cultivate awareness of what is present. This inner pause is manifested when the caregiver is completely available and present with the patient, excluding irrelevant topics and distractions.

6.2.2 Caritas Process #2

Being Authentically Present; Enabling, Sustaining, and Honoring the Faith, Hope, and Deep Belief System and the Inner Subjective Life World of Self/Other

> Hope is medicine for a soul that's sick and tired.
> – Eric Swensson

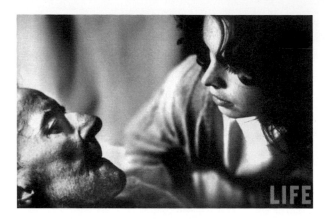

Enabling, sustaining, and honoring hope before surgery are important components of caring. Nurses do this so often that they can be unaware of the simple but profound messages of hope they offer to patients and their families. Hope is not wishful thinking or unfounded expectations for the future. It is rather about possibilities of the present moment. What can a caregiver do when people do not believe in themselves, when they doubt the possibilities? Miller and Cutshall (2001) explain that instilling faith and hope can be done in many different ways, such as:

- Patient education
- Focusing on optimistic language and the desired outcome
- Empowerment – letting the patient know they are a huge part of the healing process
- Explaining what helps and hinders the healing process

6.2.3 Caritas Process #3

Cultivation of One's Own Spiritual Practices and Transpersonal Self, Going Beyond Ego-Self

> Look closely and contemplate deeply the people and things that appear around you… All are in constant flux. Everything becomes the teacher of impermanence.
> – Seventh Dalai Lama

Watson (2008) noted that this spiritual process is a lifelong journey and a high expectation for a professional practice. For many patients and health-care providers, taking care of themselves, and focusing on healing, is a crucial step. Before surgery, many people reflect on their life, their priorities, and their sense of connectedness. One practice that can provide emotional support to a patient, who is experiencing discomfort, is to explore gratitude. This can be as simple as identifying the blessings that are concurrent with the challenge and pain. How can this become a more meaningful experience? For example, what are the small and large acts of kindness happening within the human relationships? Jean Watson (2008) describes the phenomenon of "beyond empathy" as a transpersonal experience of "connecting spirit to spirit with the other person in a given moment."

6.2.4   Caritas Process #4

Developing and Sustaining a Helping-Trusting, Authentic Caring Relationship

> The times when you are extremely vulnerable can be those when you are most open, and when you are extremely vulnerable can be where your greatest strength really lies... Suffering can, after all, teach us about compassion. If you suffer, you will know what it is like when others suffer. And if you are in a position to help others, it is through your own suffering that you will find the understanding and compassion to do so.
>   – Sogyal Rinpoche (1994)

Kaufman (1956) discusses the patient's need for presurgery emotional support. Acknowledging and reducing stress and trauma of surgery is paramount. Time needs to be sufficient for the personal connection to be made. The establishment of trust is essential between the patient and the interdisciplinary team providing preoperative and operative care. When a patient has been sufficiently prepared for the procedure, they often have a speedier and easier recovery. It is important that the patient trusts the surgeon, understands the surgery, and has faith that the outcome will be positive. The following chart illustrates the difference between curing and caring. Caring health-care professionals can make a memorable impression.

Curing	Caring
May contain healing	May occur without curing
Not always possible	Is always possible
Follows an usual or unpredictable path	Is creative and unpredictable in both process and outcome
Death is a failure to "cure" the patient	Death: an opportunity for healing, "ultimate healing"
External fixing	Inner healing

6.2.5   Caritas Process #5

Promote and Accept Positive and Negative Feelings as You Authentically Listen to Another's Story. Be Present with and Supportive of a Range of Emotions

Whatever you do, do not shut off your pain; accept your pain and remain vulnerable. However desperate you become, accept your pain as it is, because it is in fact trying to hand you a priceless gift – the chance of discovering, through spiritual practice, what lies behind sorrow.
– Sogyal Rinpoche

Before surgery, the caregiver can invite the patient to create artwork to explore their range of emotions in this challenging time. The following anecdote demonstrates a health-care professional's facilitation of an acknowledgment of the wide range of emotions that the patient experiences before surgery. This illustration elucidates how making a collage with a patient can encourage self-expression and create a space of deep listening. This is one example of how the health-care professional can utilize an art activity to promote the exploration of the spectrum of a patient's feelings.

6.2.5.1 Personalized Folder to Hold Patient's Educational Information

Materials
1. *A manila folder to hold the information about this health condition*
2. *A magazine, scissors, and glue*
3. *Open-minded presence*
    One of the first pictures the patient chooses depicts a woman holding on to a pillar. To the patient, this picture represents her holding on for strength. The patient cuts out and pastes many pictures onto the folder. As she explains the pictures, she describes the images and words she finds to represent: her endless anxiety and anguish, her sadness about how this condition that may affect her daughter, the interconnectedness she feels with her mom (who had the same genetic condition), her jealously of her sister's perfect health, etc. She and the health-care professional make eye contact while she is fully engaged in creating this piece of art and, in the midst of her angst, she says with a smile, "I am actually enjoying myself in this moment."

The patient's enjoyment of this activity demonstrates how her creative expression allows her to transcend the physical pain and experience both joy and a state of gratitude in this vulnerable time. By acknowledging the negative emotions present through art, the patient is able to open to the experience of positive emotions as well, which can support and facilitate her healing process.

6.2.6   Caritas Process #6

Use Creative Scientific Problem-Solving Methods for Caring Decision Making. Engage in the Artistry of Caring-Healing Practices

Let the beauty we love be what we do. There are hundreds of ways to kneel and kiss the ground.
– Rumi

One problem that a patient may have to deal with after surgery is the emotional and physical implications of a colostomy bag. Dwelling on these implications can contribute to pre-operation anxiety. Patients may have to deal with a different level of freedom than they are used to. They may not be able to be as active, due to the risk of the bag coming loose. Dealing with having a colostomy bag in front of the body to eliminate their waste can often elicit feelings of shame, embarrassment, and discomfort. Relaxation techniques are especially valuable in cases like this. One calming technique is the simple humming of a favorite song or of the mantra "om" while changing the colostomy bag.

6.2.7   Caritas Process #7

Share Teaching and Learning that Addresses the Individual Needs and Comprehension Styles

> Tell me and I forget, Show me and I remember, Involve me, and I understand.
>   – Chinese Proverb

Basic information can facilitate the patient and the family's ease in the presurgical situation. The best preparation includes teaching about the procedure and answering questions. Active listening and the professional team's demonstration of concern and compassion can make a tremendous difference in the patient's experience of a health crisis. As the surgeon explains the surgery, the patient has an opportunity to get to know the surgeon and build trust. Misinterpretation can be avoided if the health-care professional communicates with the patient to see if he or she actually understands. Educating patients about the surgery and recovery is most effective when tailored to the patient's own style of learning. Patients have a diversity of individual needs and comprehension styles. Some people are more visual, some learn by listening, other patients are kinesthetic learners, etc. For example, some patients may need to actually practice changing a colostomy bag to understand how to do this in a sanitary way.

6.2.8   Caritas Process #8

Create a Healing Environment for the Physical and Spiritual Self Which Respects Human Dignity

> A Buddhist Sutra states: Noble one, think of yourself as someone who is sick, Of the Dharma as the remedy, Of your spiritual friend as a skillful doctor, and of diligent practice as the way to recover.
>   – Buddhist Sutra

When a person feels seen, heard, and quintessentially important to the health-care professional, this can be soothing to their fears, anxiety, pain, and even dispel despair. The clinical setting induces stress, but if the patient feels that their needs are attended to, people may be able to relax.

In contrast, an unfocused attendant may provoke fear responses, stress, anger, or even panic. Many health-care professionals or family members are "burnt out" and end up exasperating the stress and discomfort of the patient. The caregiver may guard against such undesired states by practicing self-care for themselves when they are not with the patient. It is vital to remember to remain focused on the patient while in their room. This time can be very vulnerable, scary, and difficult for them. The human dignity of the patient is the utmost importance.

6.2.9   Caritas Process #9

Assist with Basic Physical, Emotional, and Spiritual Human Needs

> The Body is a mandala. If we look inside, it is an endless source of revelation… Without embodiment, there is no foundation from which to gain enlightenment.
> – Dr. Tsampa Ngawang

Often times, before and after surgery, basic needs are challenging for the patient. For example, after surgery, the patient may have different food and/or driving restrictions, a change in exercise regimens, and even potential modification wardrobe. The colostomy bag is a huge adjustment that the patient will need to make for a period of time. Assisting the patient with basic needs in this vulnerable time can be a very powerful way of connecting with them and providing support. Also, giving space for the patient to express themselves about their emotional and spiritual reactions can be very healing for them. One way to assist with basic physical, emotional, and spiritual human needs is to engage in and encourage ritual hand washing.

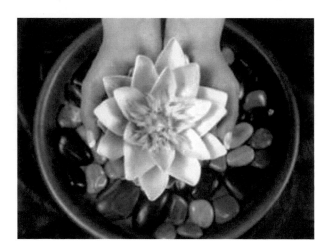

Ritual hand washing serves to:
- Wash away old experience
- Start clean and fresh
- Center in caring intention
- Honor self and others
- Reconnect to core values
- Purify sacred space for authentic presence of care

6.2.10 Caritas Process #10

Opening and Attending to Mysterious Dimensions of One's Life-Death: With Basic Physical, Emotional, and Spiritual Human Needs

> The mystery of love is greater than the mystery of death.
>   – Oscar Wilde

Prior to surgery, health-care professionals have a significant opportunity to provide caring support to the patient. Exploring the unknown existential dimensions of one's own life, death, and/or suffering can be a very powerful experience. Before their operation, the patient has an opportunity to slowdown and create time to prepare for a significant change in their body. During this time, the patient may begin to recognize what is most important to themselves and others. There is a participation in the paradox of life and death, as there are inherent risks in surgery. It is important to honor and respect the patient's inner feelings and show deep respect in this time.

6.3   Psychosocial Preparation and Coping Strategies

When approaching a surgical procedure, utilizing any of the following interventions may provide a sense of relaxation and freedom to the patient through imagining what lies beyond the surgery. There are many coping strategies than can help patients to cope with impending surgery and recovery.

6.3.1   Who Can Invite in Art and Healing?

1. Any health-care professional
2. Any friend or family member of the patient
3. The patient themselves, alone in their room
4. *No previous art experience needed*
   This is an invitation for whatever creative medium the patient wants to explore. Some presurgical art and healing possibilities include:
- Have soothing music in the background
- Write a story or poem
- Paint a T-shirt
- Play an instrument
- Make a collage
- Relaxation training
- Hypnosis
- Art makings
- Visual art
- Music
- Dance
- Poetry
- Collage

- Pain control techniques
- Positive intention/affirmations
- Preparing auditory tapes for surgery, recovery, and rehabilitation
- Journaling
- Exercise
- Yoga/meditation
- Guided imagery

6.3.2   Guided Imagery

Guided imagery is a directed deliberate visualization that is similar to daydreaming. This technique guides the inner world of personal imagery. This coping strategy can be utilized prior to surgery. Practicing guided imagery once or twice a day for several weeks prior to surgery can make a difference with pain and decrease the number of inpatient days after the surgery. It is a technique of accessing an altered state of relaxation. Since surgery creates a stressful situation, guided imagery helps with general anxiety and promotes feelings of balance, peace, and optimism. Guided imagery can heighten feelings of love and safety, which can increase the serotonin levels and create an inner feeling of calm.

According to Tusek et al. (1997), guided imagery has been shown to:
- Relieve anxiety and stress pre- and post-procedure
- Reduce pain
- Improve sleep
- Speed recovery
- Reduce side effects
- Reduce blood loss
- Decrease complications from anesthesia

6.3.3   Guided Imagery and Psychosocial Preparation for Surgery

Surgery can result in loss of control, where a person feels more like a victim than an active participant in their own care. Anxiety and fear of the unknown and of pain increases a person's pain perception and side effects of pain medicines and effect healing. These stresses also result in longer postoperative recovery and suppressed immune system. There are many things patients can do to prepare for surgery that improve outcome including guided imagery, making art, relaxation, and positive expectations.

Guided imagery uses images in the mind or imagination to effect psychological and physiological states. The patient uses a CD or mp3 to picture mental images in a state of focused concentration. This produces relaxation and physical and emotional well-being. It has been shown to help people strengthen their immune system and enhance their healing.

Tusek et al. (1997) and others at the Cleveland Clinic looked at guided imagery with 130 patients undergoing colorectal surgery. The control group received standard surgical care and the experiment group used a guided imagery tape with soft, soothing music and words which took them on an inner imagination journey to a place that was safe and secure. Patients listened to the tape two times a day, for 3 days, before the operation and for 6 days after. During surgery and in the recovery room, they were given a CD with the music.

The experimental group who used guided imagery had less pain and anxiety before and after surgery. For example, colostomy patients who used guided imagery needed only half the amount of narcotic pain medication and bowel function returned much more quickly.

Guided imagery is the basic tool to allow the mind to concentrate and hold images that promote relaxation and healing.

There are easy steps to guided imagery that are easy to learn and teach patients to prepare for surgery:

1. *Breathing*: Make yourself comfortable. You can be sitting down or laying down. Loosen tight clothing; uncross your legs and arms. Close your eyes. Let your breathing slowdown. Take several deep breaths. Let your abdomen rise as you breathe in and fall as you let your deep breath out. As you breathe in and out, you will become more and more relaxed. You may experience feelings of tingling, buzzing, or relaxation. If you do, let those feelings increase. You may feel heaviness or lightness; you may feel your boundaries loosening and your edges softening. As you breathe in, let yourself fill with energy. As you breathe out, let whatever you want to leave your body exit with your breath.

2. *Relaxation*: Now let yourself relax. Let your feet relax; let your legs relax. Let the feelings of relaxation spread upward to your thighs and pelvis. Let your pelvis open and relax. Now let your abdomen relax, let your belly expand, and do not hold it in anymore. Now let your chest relax; let your heartbeat and breathing take place by themselves. Let your arms relax and your hands relax. Now let your neck relax, your head, and your face. Let your eyes relax; see a horizon and blackness for a moment. Let these feelings of relaxation spread throughout your body.

3. *Deepening*: Let your relaxation deepen. If you wish, you can count your breaths and let your relaxation deepen with each breath. You can picture going deeper in a cave, a walk into a forest that goes down a long path, an elevator with floor numbers, and a long hallway, whatever seems most at home for you. As you deepen, you can allow your body to expand. It can expand to one third larger that its usual size. As you expand, let space appear between you cells. Let the space fill with energy. Let the energy come up into you from the earth and down into you from the sky. As you breathe in, let the energy grow; as you breathe out, let the energy remain high.

4. *The content*: In your mind's eye, see yourself the night before the surgery resting peacefully and calmly in bed. See yourself feel as safe and comfortable, sleeping soundly. Know that you will trust your doctors who have done this many times and know you will have an easy day during the surgery. See yourself, cheerful, talking to the staff, and seeing beauty and love around you. In your mind's eye, know that nothing will bother you. You will be in a calm, relaxed state of trust. Know that in the morning, you won't want to eat or drink

anything, so that all of your body functions will be at rest. You body will not be hungry or thirsty. Now see yourself leaving your room and going to surgery. As you go, let yourself drift to a safe place that is your home inside your mind. It can be a place you love, a meadow, beach, mountain, a place you feel perfectly at home. From the time you leave your room, until you return from the recovery room, you should simply enjoy your special place and completely ignore anything that people say unless you are spoken to directly by name. Know that when the anesthesia is started, you will feel absolutely no pain. If you hear sounds, simply ignore them because you will be feeling no pain, and you will be in your special safe place of enhanced protection and grace. Know that you will get as much air as you need through the small tube in the back of your throat. If you want to, you can see the hands of your surgeon working adeptly and skillfully. Throughout surgery, your breathing will be even and relaxed. Later, see yourself being moved to a stretcher and taken to the recovery room. See yourself gradually awakening just as you do from natural sleep, relaxed and refreshed. See yourself waking up remarkably comfortable, with a good appetite, and your normal bladder and bowel functions coming back quickly. Know that whatever you need for comfort will be supplied, and your body will heal rapidly and perfectly.

5. *Grounding and closing*: When you are ready, return to the room where you are doing the exercise. Press your backside down on the place you are sitting or lying. Press you feet down hard on the floor or ground. First, move your feet and then move your hands. Move them around and experience the feeling of the movement. Press your feet down harder onto the floor, feel the grounding, feel the pressure on the bottom of your feet, and feel the solidity of the earth. Feel your backside on the chair; feel your weight pressing downward. Now open your eyes. Look around you. Stand up and stretch, move your body, and feel it move.

6. *Final instructions for healing*: You are back; you can carry the experience of the exercise outward to your life. You will feel stronger and be able to see deeper. You will be in a healing state. You can do this exercise whenever you wish; as you read the book, the visions you have will deepen. You may discover that the physical and emotional relaxation becomes faster and easier the more times you practice guided imagery.

6.3.4 Spiritual Issues

We are not just physical beings having a spiritual experience; rather we are spiritual beings having a physical experience.
    – Teilhard de Chardin

Prayer and belief in a higher power have great meaning for some patients. Incorporating spiritual techniques such as prayer into the psychological preparation can have benefits such as these:

• Provide the patient with some comfort in the face of their illness, fears, or surgery.

- Help provide a sense of meaning and purpose beyond the other explanations provided.
- Combining prayer or meditation can assist in the relaxation response which can contribute positively to the patients overall feelings of wellness.

Caregivers attempting to incorporate spirituality may face resistance from the patient or from one or more family members. When incorporating spirituality into preoperative care, caregivers must respect the belief systems of the patient and his or her attending family members.

The following anecdote from one of the authors' experiences illustrates how referencing spirituality before surgery impacts family members in very different ways. Utilizing spiritual language creates soothing and connecting opportunities for two family members. Alternatively, spiritual discussion brings up resistance in two other family members.

In the surgery waiting room, a daughter of the patient receives a text, "Sending strength and peace to your mom and her body. Sending focus and loving kindness to the health care professionals working with her." This daughter starts to cry in gratitude and actually visualizes sending that beautiful prayer to the doctors ... Although there is no "right thing" to say at times like these, that text seemed like the most fitting and valuable words for this family member to receive in these scary and helpless moments.

She reads this text out loud to her sisters and father. One sister looks up in surprise, because in that very moment, she had been texting a religious friend, asking for prayers for their mom. The sisters felt so connected through this synchronous reaching out through spirituality and prayer.

However, the father of these sisters (the loving husband of the patient) is a physician who was also having a very hard time with his wife going into surgery. In response to hearing this text, with tears in his eyes, he exclaimed, "I do not want to hear about spirituality right now!" He then proceeded to talk with his medical colleague to scientifically discuss further implications of the surgery.

The patient also felt infringed upon by this daughter's frequent mention of spiritual adages. The patient said in a strong tone of voice, "Your focus on spirituality does not help me."

This excerpt exemplifies the importance of choosing words carefully, especially when people are in such a vulnerable condition. After this experience, language was approached in a more careful way.

The spiritually oriented daughter and her mother, the patient, laughed and smiled as they listened to music and worked on making a photo album gift together. There was no verbal mention of what a spiritual experience this felt like to the daughter. The meaningful time they spent making gifts together was certainly full of serenity, bonding, and gratitude. These are all spiritual values her daughter holds, and although she was feeling a very deep sacredness within these moments, the daughter of course did not explicitly point this out. She had realized that with her mom, the overt mentioning of spirituality brought up uneasiness.

In contrast, she also realized spiritual language with her sister brought them closer together. Different family members certainly had diverse reactions to internal and external experiences of spirituality in this pre- and postsurgical time.

6.3.5 Humor

Another anecdote from this experience acknowledges how humor can be uplifting and provide opportunities of connection with the patient. Humor can bring joy and quality time to the presurgical experience. However, humor can also be inappropriate and offensive when the humor is not perceived as respectful or if humor is interjected at an inappropriate time.

Humor, although it has been said to be the best medicine, was a bit touch and go with this patient. At first, the patient smiled about the lighthearted jokes that were made by her family members about the upcoming surgery. She even laughed a couple of times and seemed to appreciate how the humor of those around her lightened her heavy mood.

At one point, the doctor cautioned that "laughter, some movements, and going to the bathroom" might be painful. When her daughter exclaimed, "OMG ("Oh My Gosh")! How can one live without laughing, moving, or using the bathroom?!" The patient actually (LOL) "laughed out loud" in response to this.

However, at a certain point, the integration of humor in this very serious time was too much for the patient. She crossed her arms and loudly announced, "This is NOT FUNNY!"

At times, the tension in the room was broken by the laughter. The mood changed dramatically because of the humor. However, it is important to make sure that the humor is appropriate for the circumstances and personal preferences of the patient.

Conclusion

In summary, this chapter outlines the significance and importance of psychosocial preparation before surgery. The ten Caritas Processes are presented to help guide caring practices. Examples and narratives are provided throughout this chapter to give insight into the integration of available interventions. Integrating creativity and spirituality, whether or not this is explicitly verbalized, can promote healing and offer comfort to patients and their families. Health-care professionals that meet their patient where they are at by recognizing their humanness and allowing space for their difficult emotions such as fear or stress can make a tremendous difference in the well-being of the patient. Caring is different than curing.

References

Kaufman W (1956) The physician's role in the preparation of a patient for surgery. In: Cantor AJ, Foxe AN (eds) Psychosomatic aspects of surgery. Grune and Stratton, New York, pp 1–2, (2) Dyk, R. B., and Sutherland, A. M.: Adaptation

Miller J, Cutshall S (2001) The art of being a healing presence: a guide to those in caring relationships. Willowgreen Publishing, Fort Wayne

Rinpoche S (1994) The Tibetan book of living and dying: a new spiritual classic from one of the foremost interpreters of Tibetan Buddhism to the west. HarperCollins Publishers, San Francisco, California

Tusek DL et al (1997) Guided imagery: a significant advance in the care of patients undergoing elective colorectal surgery. Dis Colon Rectum 40:172–178

Watson J (2008) Nursing the philosophy and science of caring Rev. edn. University Press of Colorado, Boulder

Prehabilitation

7

Lawrence Tan

Take Home Pearls

- Exercise and improving physical capacity is beneficial for the elderly across a wide spectrum of medical conditions.
- Prehabilitation is the process of enhancing the functional capacity of an individual to enable him or her to withstand a stressful event.
- In the context of surgery, prehabilitation has been described to be the use of exercise training preoperatively to improve postoperative outcomes.
- A more holistic approach including attention to the physical ability, nutrition, and psychosocial needs is likely to lead to more success.

7.1 Introduction

It is well recognised that exercise is beneficial for the elderly across many medical conditions. Studies have demonstrated a relationship between regular exercise and improvements in outcome measures such as coronary artery disease, hypertension, type 2 diabetes mellitus, stroke disease and osteoporosis. The American College of Sports Medicine and the American Heart Association published recommendations for physical activity in older adults in 2007. These recommendations include

L. Tan
Department of Geriatric Medicine,
Geriatric Surgery Service, Khoo Teck
Puat Hospital, Alexandra Health,
Singapore, Singapore
e-mail: lawrencetanwm@yahoo.com

K.-Y. Tan (ed.), *Colorectal Cancer in the Elderly*,
DOI 10.1007/978-3-642-29883-7_7, © Springer-Verlag Berlin Heidelberg 2013

incorporating moderate-intensity aerobic activity, developing muscle strength with resistance training and flexibility/balance exercises.

While factors such as chronological age, a reduction in the ability to respond to stress, frailty and co-morbid illnesses influence postoperative complications, there is also an association between physical fitness and outcomes following surgery. Patients who are less fit with poor baseline physical performance capacity tend to have a higher incidence of perioperative complications. Cardiopulmonary exercise testing can be useful in identifying patients at increased risk of adverse outcomes following non-cardiopulmonary surgery.

Since physical fitness plays a role in postoperative outcomes, improving physical fitness preoperatively should lead to better outcomes. Unfortunately, there is currently little evidence to suggest that exercise training preoperatively may improve postoperative outcomes in the elderly.

Previous studies have explored the restoration of function in disabled elderly patients through rehabilitation after an acute medical illness such as a stroke or after surgical procedures. There have been few studies evaluating strategies aimed at the prevention of functional decline in elderly patients who have not had an acute illness or injury or undergone surgery.

The process of enhancing the functional capacity of the individual to enable him or her to withstand a stressful event has been termed 'prehabilitation'.

In a study published in 2002, Gill et al. conducted a randomised clinical trial of a home-based programme designed to prevent functional decline in a high-risk group of frail elderly persons living at home. In this trial, 188 frail elderly persons aged 75 years or older who were living at home were randomly assigned to undergo a 6-month, home-based intervention programme that focused on improving physical function which included muscle strength, balance and mobility or to undergo an educational programme (control). The primary outcome was the change between baseline function and 3, 7 and 12 months in the score on a disability scale based on eight activities of daily living.

Participants in the intervention group were visited at home by a physical therapist an average of 16 times over a 6-month period. Recommended interventions included progressive resistance exercises using elastic bands, training in the proper use of assistive devices, removal of hazardous obstacles (e.g. loose rugs, cords, clutter), instruction on safe techniques for facilitating activities, improvement in lighting, repair of walking surfaces and installation of adaptive equipment in the bathroom.

The control group received 6 monthly home visits by a health educator where general practices promoting good health such as proper nutrition, sleep hygiene and management of medications were reviewed. The results showed that, compared to the control group, participants in the intervention group experienced less disability at 7 and 12 months. The benefits of the intervention were mostly among participants with moderate frailty. Persons with severe disability experienced worsening disability over time, despite the intervention. The reason for this is unclear.

7.2   Effect of Prehabilitation on Postoperative Outcomes After Hip and Knee Replacement Surgery

Apart from a few studies demonstrating the beneficial effects of preoperative exercise training on postoperative outcomes following hip and knee replacement surgery, most have tended to show little significant change in outcome measures.

A study by D'Lima et al., published in 1996, compared the effects of preoperative physical therapy which included muscle strengthening exercises as well as cardiovascular conditioning exercises on total knee replacement outcomes. Thirty patients were randomised to 1 of 3 groups. Group 1 was the control group, Group 2 participated in a programme to strengthen upper and lower limbs and Group 3 participated in a cardiovascular conditioning programme. All 3 groups showed significant improvement postoperatively as measured by the Hospital for Special Surgery Knee Rating Scale, the Arthritis Impact Measurement Scale and the Quality of Well-Being Measurement Scale. However, neither type of preoperative exercise added to the degree of improvement after surgery at any of the postoperative evaluations.

In a study by Rodgers et al. (1998), ten patients completed 6 weeks of physical therapy prior to total knee arthroplasty and another 10 patients served as controls. Subjects were tested at baseline, before surgery, 6 weeks after surgery and 3 months after surgery using various parameters such as walking speed, thigh circumference, isokinetic knee flexion and extension testing and computed tomography scanning to determine cross-sectional muscle area. Physical therapy produced modest gains in isokinetic flexion strength but no difference in extension strength. The decrease in isokinetic strength after surgery was unaffected by preoperative physical therapy. Muscle area did not decrease significantly for the physical therapy group, but it did decrease for the control group after surgery.

Beaupre et al. (2004) looked at the effectiveness of a preoperative exercise/education programme on functional recovery, health-related quality of life (HRQOL), health service utilisation and costs following primary total knee arthroplasty. One hundred and thirty-one patients were randomised to either a control or treatment group 6 weeks before surgery. Patients in the treatment group underwent a 4-week exercise/education programme before surgery. No differences were seen in knee measurements (range of movement and strength), pain, function or HRQOL between the 2 groups following the intervention programme or at any postoperative measurement point. Patients in the treatment group used fewer postoperative rehabilitation services and stayed for a shorter time in hospital than the control group, but these differences did not attain statistical significance.

One of the few studies showing beneficial effects of preoperative exercise therapy in patients undergoing hip/knee replacement surgery was published by Rooks et al. in 2006. In this study, 108 men and women scheduled for either total hip or total knee arthroplasty were randomised to a 6-week exercise or education (control) intervention prior to surgery. Outcome measurements, which included questionnaires and performance measures, were measured preoperatively, immediately postoperatively, 8 weeks and 26 weeks post-surgery. Among the hip replacement patients, the exercise intervention was associated with improvements in the questionnaire data in the intervention group. No significant differences were noted in the knee replacement group. Muscle strength increased in both the knee and hip replacement patients in the intervention group.

7.3   Effect of Prehabilitation on Postoperative Outcomes After Colorectal Surgery

A randomised controlled trial of prehabilitation in patients undergoing colorectal surgery was published by Carli et al. in 2010, where the extent to which a structured prehabilitation regimen of stationary cycling and strengthening optimised recovery of functional walking capacity after surgery was compared with a simpler regimen of walking and breathing exercises. In this study, 112 patients were randomised to either a bike and strengthening regimen (bike/strengthening group) or a simpler walking and breathing regimen (walk/breathing group). The mean time to surgery available for prehabilitation was 52 days and the follow-up was for 10 weeks after surgery. The primary outcome measure was functional walking capacity measured by the 6-min Walk Test. This test evaluates the capacity of a person to maintain a moderate level of walking for a period of time.

There were no differences between the groups in mean functional walking capacity over the prehabilitation period or at postoperative follow-up. However, a greater proportion of patients assigned to the walk/breathing group recovered functional walking capacity postoperatively compared to those assigned to the bike/strengthening group.

More recently, a reanalysis of the trial data was carried out to determine the extent to which physical function could be improved with either prehabilitation intervention and to identify variables associated with a positive response. Of 95 patients who completed a prehabilitation programme while awaiting colorectal surgery, 33% improved their physical function, 38% remained the same and 29% deteriorated. Patients randomised to the walk/breathing group were more likely to improve compared to the bike/strengthening group. At postoperative follow-up, those who improved during prehabilitation were more likely to have recovered to baseline functional walking capacity compared to those who did not change or who deteriorated. Patients who deteriorated while awaiting surgery were at particular risk for more serious surgical complications.

Improved preoperative functional capacity remained a predictor of recovery after adjusting for variables such as age, diagnosis, complications and baseline physical capacity. The analysis suggests that a prehabilitation programme based on walking and breathing exercises can improve functional exercise capacity in patients awaiting colorectal surgery, and this improvement is associated with improved postoperative recovery.

7.4 Effect of Prehabilitation on Postoperative Outcomes After Spinal Surgery

In randomised clinical trial conducted by Nielsen PR from 2003 to 2005, 60 patients were assigned to either prehabilitation (exercise programme) and early rehabilitation or to standard care. The outcome measures included postoperative hospital stay, complications and patient satisfaction.

The patients in the prehabilitation group had faster improvement in function, shorter hospital stays and higher satisfaction, without more complications or pain.

7.5 Effect of Preoperative Inspiratory Muscle Training on Postoperative Outcomes After Cardiac or Major Vascular Surgery

Pulmonary complications after cardiac surgery are a major cause of postoperative morbidity and mortality. Respiratory muscle weakness may contribute to the postoperative pulmonary complications. Several studies have used inspiratory muscle training as the intervention in elderly patients undergoing coronary artery bypass grafting or abdominal aortic aneurysm surgery.

Hulzebos et al. (2006) evaluated the effect of preoperative inspiratory muscle training on the incidence of postoperative pulmonary complications in high-risk patients scheduled for elective coronary artery bypass grafting. The results showed that preoperative inspiratory muscle training reduced the incidence of postoperative pulmonary complications and duration of postoperative hospitalisation.

In a study by Dronkers et al. (2008), 20 high-risk patients undergoing elective abdominal aneurysm surgery were randomly assigned to receive either preoperative inspiratory muscle training or usual care. Outcome measures included atelectasis, inspiratory muscle strength and vital capacity.

Fewer patients in the intervention group developed atelectasis compared to the control group, but the incidence of postoperative pulmonary complications was not significantly reduced.

7.6 Prehabilitation in the Context of Geriatric Surgery

The failure of available data to show consistent benefit in their study cohorts is somewhat puzzling. Indeed, if time is taken to improve physical and cardiorespiratory function prior to surgery, why would it be unsuccessful? It is our opinion that this phenomenon may be secondary to the lack of a holistic approach to prehabilitation. While trying to conduct very scientific experiments, many of the described studies had failed to consider the patient as a whole. It should be realised that prehabilitation is not just about improving one aspect of the patient; rather the approach should be more holistic and the aim should be to improve the entire well-being of the patient. It cannot be just about physical aspects, psychosocial and nutritional aspects are equally important.

Our suggested framework for prehabilitation for elderly surgical patients aims to address the various facets important to the entire well-being of the patient. The key elements include:

- Education and empowerment of the patient in their own recovery process
- Attention to psychosocial needs
- Cardiopulmonary strengthening
- Walking and mobilising
- Muscle strengthening
- Attention to nutrition
- Attention to activities of daily living

The delivery of such a holistic process can only be facilitated by a transdisciplinary team. Constant review, reassessment and setting of goals with open communication between the team, patient and carers are the cornerstones of successful care delivery. Table 7.1 shows the Khoo Teck Puat Hospital Geriatric Surgery Programme prehabilitation goal setting in the various elements of our programme.

The duration and time frame for prehabilitation has to be tailored to the urgency of the surgery. Prehabilitation is most ideally done in the comfort of the patients' own homes. However, day centres are also viable options. Inpatient prehabilitation should only be performed for the very frail.

Table 7.1 Khoo Teck Puat Hospital Geriatric Surgery Programme: prehabilitation goal setting

Component	Initial assessment	One week after prehabilitation		Two weeks after prehabilitation		Target
Education and compliance	Understands disease and indication for surgery	Patient understands disease and indication for surgery	Yes ☐ No ☐	Patient understands disease and indication for surgery	Yes ☐ No ☐	Patient understands disease and indication for surgery
	Knows what to expect	Patient knows what to expect	Yes ☐ No ☐	Patient knows what to expect	Yes ☐ No ☐	Patient knows what to expect
	Preparation for operation	Patient knows what to do	Yes ☐ No ☐	Patient knows what to do	Yes ☐ No ☐	Patient knows what to do
Weight change	Current weight:	No weight loss Weight loss ≤5% Weight loss >5%	☐ ☐ ☐	No weight loss Weight loss ≤5% Weight loss >5%	☐ ☐ ☐	No weight loss over past 2 weeks
Dietary intake	Usual intake:	Achieved 100% of dietary requirement 5 in 7 days	Yes ☐ No ☐	Achieved 100% of dietary requirement 5 in 7 days	Yes ☐ No ☐	Achieved 100% of dietary requirement 5 in 7 days
Chair to stand	No of reps:	No of reps: Significant improvement (>10%) Good improvement (5–10%) No/little improvement (<5%)	☐ ☐ ☐	No of reps: Significant improvement (>10%) Good improvement (5–10%) No/little improvement (<5%)	☐ ☐ ☐	No of reps: Achieved significant improvement (>10%)

Table 7.1 (continued)

Component	Initial assessment	One week after prehabilitation		Two weeks after prehabilitation		Target
10-m walk test	No of steps:	No of steps:		No of steps:		No of steps:
		Significant improvement (>3%)	☐	Significant improvement (>3%)	☐	Significant improvement (>3%)
		Good improvement (1–3%)	☐	Good improvement (1–3%)	☐	
		No/little improvement (<1%)	☐	No/little improvement (<1%)	☐	
	Time taken (s):	Time taken (s):		Time taken (s):		Time taken (s):
		Significant improvement (>3%)	☐	Significant improvement (>3%)	☐	Significant improvement (>3%)
		Good improvement (1–3%)	☐	Good improvement (1–3%)	☐	
		No/little improvement (<1%)	☐	No/little improvement (<1%)	☐	

Conclusion

The results from the limited number of trials in prehabilitation are promising but inconsistent. It is likely that only a more holistic team-based approach can afford better results. Prehabilitation processes in elderly surgical patients remain a work in progress.

References

Beaupre LA, Lier D, Davies DM, Johnston DB (2004) The effect of a preoperative exercise and education program on functional recovery, health related quality of life, and health service utilization following primary total knee arthroplasty. J Rheumatol 31(6):1166–1173

Carli F, Charlebois P, Stein B, Feldman L, Zavorsky G, Kim DJ, Scott S, Mayo NE (2010) Randomised clinical trial of prehabilitation in colorectal surgery. Br J Surg 97(8):1187–1197

D'Lima DD, Colwell CW Jr, Morris BA, Hardwick ME, Kozin F (1996) The effect of preoperative exercise on total knee replacement outcomes. Clin Orthop Relat Res 326:174–182

Dronkers J, Veldman A, Hoberg E, van der Waal C, van Meeteren N (2008) Prevention of pulmonary complications after upper abdominal surgery by preoperative intensive inspiratory muscle training: a randomized controlled pilot study. Clin Rehabil 22(2):134–142

Gill TM, Baker DI, Gottschalk M, Peduzzi PN, Allore H, Byers A (2002) A program to prevent functional decline in physically frail, elderly persons who live at home. N Engl J Med 347:1068–1074

Hulzebos EH, van Meeteren NL, van den Buijs BJ, de Bie RA, Brutel de la Riviere A, Helders PJ (2006) Feasibility of preoperative inspiratory muscle training in patients undergoing coronary artery bypass surgery with a high risk of postoperative pulmonary complications: a randomized controlled pilot study. Clin Rehabil 20(11):949–959

Rodgers JA, Garvin KL, Walker CW, Morford D, Urban J, Bedard J (1998) Preoperative physical therapy in primary total knee arthroplasty. J Arthroplasty 13(4):414–421

Rooks DS, Huang J, Bierbaum BE, Bolus SA, Rubano J, Connolly CE, Alpert S, Iversen MD, Katz JN (2006) Effect of preoperative exercise on measures of functional status in men and women undergoing total hip and knee arthroplasty. Arthritis Rheum 55(5):700–708

Transdisciplinary Care for Elderly Surgical Patients

8

Kok-Yang Tan and Phyllis Xiu-Zhuang Tan

Take Home Pearls

- Elderly surgical patients demand more coordinated holistic care.
- Multidisciplinary care can still give rise to fragmented delivery of care.
- Transdisciplinary care is an evolution of multidisciplinary care with heightened communication and coordination.
- Transdisciplinary care demands modifications in the roles of the team members.

8.1 Background

The elderly population is increasing. With this come increased responsibilities for surgeons who face an increasing number of elderly patients. Management of the elderly surgical patient is complex owing to higher incidence of comorbidities and reduced functional reserves. Many of these complexities go beyond the boundaries of a surgeon's expertise, and team approach must take precedence.

8.2 Multidisciplinary Care

Multidisciplinary care was a buzzword of the 1990s with an increased recognition that the input from various physicians and allied health professionals would benefit patients over compartmentalized medicine. In surgery, most centers have adopted a

K.-Y. Tan (✉) • P.X.-Z. Tan
Department of Surgery,
Geriatric Surgery Service,
Khoo Teck Puat Hospital, Alexandra Health,
Singapore
e-mail: kokyangtan@gmail.com

K.-Y. Tan (ed.), *Colorectal Cancer in the Elderly*,
DOI 10.1007/978-3-642-29883-7_8, © Springer-Verlag Berlin Heidelberg 2013

multidisciplinary approach for major surgery to varying extents. This approach is, however, often not optimal. In the traditional multidisciplinary approach that many units are practicing, members of the multidisciplinary team have individual roles and give separate input on the patient based on their own education and expertise. For the surgical patient, the surgeon often becomes the gatekeeper determining who should be involved in this team for each patient. Communication among the team members is often limited to specified team meetings, if any, at all. This model of treatment gives rise to fragmentation, incoordination and care for patients still remained in treatment silos and compartmentalization remained. Furthermore, patients are seldom involved in the care process and are not empowered to look after themselves.

8.3   Transdisciplinary Care

The concept of transdisciplinary care has been described for sometime already mostly by our nursing counterparts (Reilly 2001). It was first proposed as a model for educating cerebral palsy-inflicted children (Walker and Avant 1995). Transdisciplinary care is a product of evolution from multidisciplinary care to a more integrated, collaborative, and less compartmentalized approach. This model became recognized as suitable for healthcare delivery and has since been proposed as a superior practice model for nurse practitioners (Walker and Avant 1995; Wilson 1996; Caramanica and Anderson 2001). Transdisciplinary approach has unfortunately to date been seldom described in surgical patients.

A collaborative transdisciplinary model of care aims to break all boundaries and is in part facilitated by the current technology and information revolution. Transdisciplinary care dispenses of hierarchy and communication is free flowing and ongoing, it is coordinated, it is seamless, it aims to improve constantly, and transdisciplinary care is more involved (Mitchell 2005; Emmons et al. 2008). The main aim of transdisciplinary model is to provide an integrated and coordinated assessment and care plan with an ultimate unified management.

The concept of a transdisciplinary approach in surgical patients is perhaps the most applicable in elderly patients. In order to provide the most holistic care to an elderly surgical patient, numerous interacting factors need to be considered. There are physiological changes associated with aging. Elderly patients have a higher incidence of comorbidity and are more complex than most younger patients (Christmas et al. 2006); furthermore, their functional reserves are poorer reducing the margin of error that can be allowed in the patients' management. Chronic pain may also lead to immobility and reduced functional status further increasing the risk of surgery.

There are also numerous psychosocial issues that may come to a critical point in the setting of major surgery. The incidence of psychogeriatric problems and cognitive impairment creates challenge for the provider. There are many elderly who live alone and face isolation and loneliness, and there are also significant financial implications.

All these above issues may increase stress to the patient, and together with the need for polypharmacy to treat their chronic illnesses, there is an increased risk of malnutrition and hygiene associated problems.

Surgical management should aim not only to reduce morbidity and mortality in this group of patients, but more importantly, their postoperative functional status should be addressed aggressively so as to preserve the independence of these patients. Indeed, in an elderly patient, failure to address all these issues may have a negative impact on the patients' outcomes.

8.4   Implementing Transdisciplinary Care

Implementing changes from multidisciplinary care to transdisciplinary care in elderly surgery may be a daunting process particular in institutions deep-seated in the practice of multidisciplinary care. Barriers to implementation include lack of manpower, lack of understanding of the education and expertise among different healthcare professionals, lack of buying-in among the players, turf issues, and also a lack of a patient-centered culture (Reilly 2001). In creating a transdisciplinary surgical team, it is important to take pointers from our nursing colleagues who have been the main champions of these changes (Fig. 8.1).

Reilly quite aptly explained the requirement of the following premises for transdisciplinary care: role extension, role enrichment, role expansion, role release, and role support. Role extension involves a constant improvement in the knowledge of one's discipline, attaining security in one's role and responsibility, thus resolving turf issues (Reilly 2001). Role enrichment involves the acquiring of knowledge and understanding of other disciplines on the team through excellent communication and collaboration. Role expansion represents the next step in this evolution where each member of a discipline educates the others on his or her own expertise though meetings and reviews. Through these measures, role release can be effected with blurring of the traditional disciplinary boundaries, and these transdisciplinary boundaries should then be supported through encouragement and feedback from other team members (role support). Constant sharing of knowledge, expertise, and responsibilities across the disciplines with cross-training and flexibility define a transdisciplinary approach (Fig. 8.2).

A change in mind-set should be nurtured with an increased understanding that problems in elderly surgical patients are not mutually exclusive and that surgical care requires a much more holistic approach rather than just addressing physical issues, especially for the elderly. Cause and effect relationships need to be considered on a much broader basis and require views from different perspectives.

The Geriatric Surgery Service of our institution embraces transdisciplinary care in the management of our elderly surgical patients. Figure 8.3 illustrates the interactions of the team centered on the patient. Service make-up, strategies, and philosophies are reported in a recent article. Through this approach, we have been able to

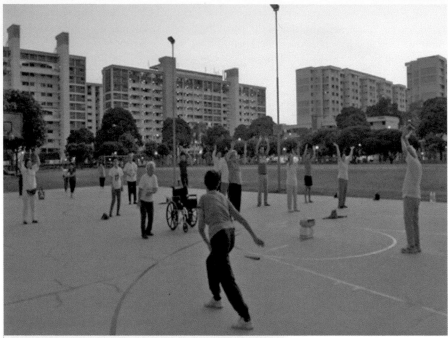

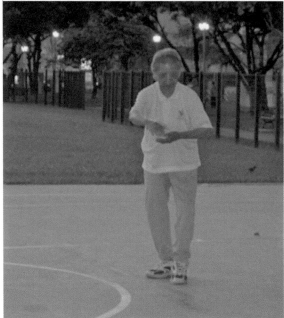

Fig. 8.1 This 82 year old Tai Chi master's main goal for cancer treatment was to be able to continue teaching after treatment and she managed to achieve it

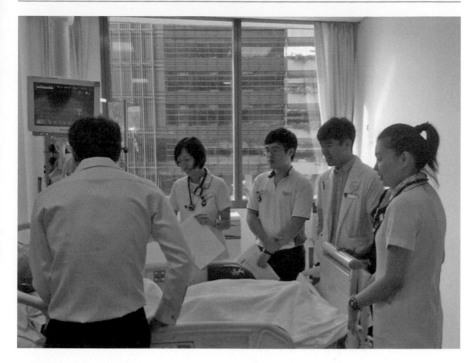

Fig. 8.2 Transdisciplinary rounds facilitate interdisciplinary communication and discussions that are vital to this model

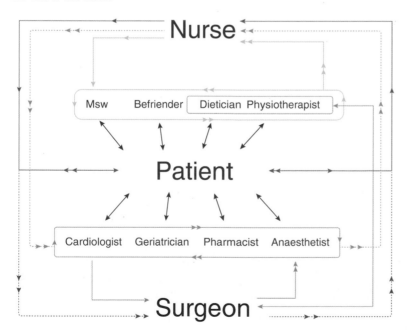

Fig. 8.3 Communication pathways in the Alexandra Health Geriatric Surgery Service transdisciplinary model of care

Table 8.1 The role and actions of the team members in the multi-faceted perioperative care of an elderly colorectal surgery patient

Time	Surgeon	Nurse	Pharmacist	Geriatrician	Anaesthetist	Cardiologist	MSW	PT	Dietician	Befriender
Diagnosis	Counselled patient and family on diagnosis and surgical management plans	Activated team after patient agreed for surgery								
Pre-op	Identified goals and planned surgery including contingency plans with patient and family. Main goal is a return to independence after curative surgery	Education was done on what to expect and to ensure patient understands the need for compliance post operatively. Identified patient to be staying alone most of the time. Visits grand daughter with public transport. A continued active lifestyle is vital. Stoma care training with appliances was conducted for confidence building and to allay anxiety. Communication with MSW includes: Discharge planning, Care upon discharge, Stoma care	Reconciled medication to prevent poly-pharmacy and drug interaction	Directed work-up for adrenal lesion with conclusion of incidentaloma. Reassessed patient thoroughly including medical risk factors for post operative delirium	Educated patient and established pain relief measures. Planned medications in accordance to comorbidities and prevention of post operative delirium	Optimised cardiac function and blood pressure control with medication	Performed socioeconomic assessment. Discussed with nurse and planned for smooth discharge process	Assessed baseline function. Established rehabilitation plan with input from surgeon. Education done. Exercises started	Planned nutritional support effectively in relation to physical and biochemistry status	Established rapport with patient and communication was carried out with nurse to better understand patient's social status

Intra-op	Meticulous surgery with careful dissection All pelvic nerves preserved Blood loss <200mls Minimal lines used to facilitate early mobilisation			Epidural analgesia Careful control of blood pressure Careful prevention of hypothermia	
POD1	Updated family of progress. Assessed physiological and clinical status Initiated oral analgesia from op day to minimize usage of morphine Initiated feeding tolerated	Coordinated medical and nursing care of patient Ensured patient receives adequate nutrition as recommended by dietitian in accordance to order from surgeon	Reviewed medications and made recommendation line with status of patient's progress	Pain assessment & management of fluid balance Blood tests were ordered to ensure electrolytes balance Ensured minimal flutuations in blood pressure	Daily review to optimize lung function and progressive ambulatory rehabilitation
POD2	Daily assessment and review of care plan according to progress of patient	Reinforced on pre-op education and surgeon's management plan		Pain assessment	
POD3	Lines were removed from POD3	Discontinued epidural analgesia			Provided "food-for-soul" through chats and walks

(continued)

Table 8.1 (continued)

Time	Surgeon	Nurse	Pharmacist	Geriatrician	Anaesthetist	Cardiologist	MSW	PT	Dietician	Befriender
POD4	Titrated fluid management according to ileostomy output	Maintained communication with family on update of management plans	Reviewed medications before discharge	Medication adjusted for BP control		Assessed need for further cardiovascular optimisation	Discussed with patient and family to coordinate for rehabilitation hospital application as suggested	Assessed progress of rehabilitation and discussed benefits to community hospital for short term rehab	Nutritional supplements adjusted in accordance to oral intake to meet calorie needs	
POD5	Progressive escalation of diet Constant updates to family	Caregiver training for stoma and wound care						Continuation of rehabilitation till discharge		
POD6	Finalised discharge plan	Communicates with Rehab hospital to ensure continuity of care							Dietary education done	
POD7	Discharged to Rehabilitation Hospital, independent with activities of daily living at this point									

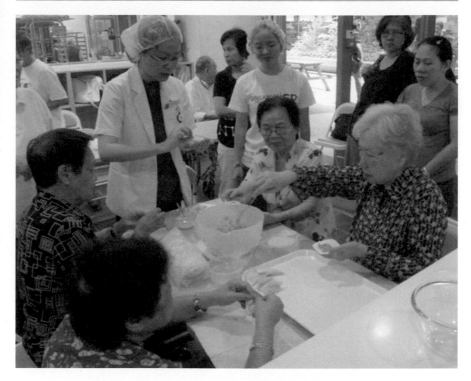

Fig. 8.4 Activities are organized to help patients continue with activities at home

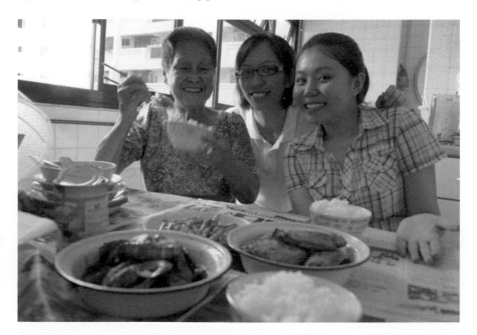

Fig. 8.5 Visits are made to ensure continued functional independence and social integration

achieve lower perioperative complication rates and a return to premorbid functional status in nearly 85% of our patients within 6 weeks for major colorectal surgeries. The service was also able to achieve sustained improvement with each successive patient managed.

8.5   Case Study of Transdisciplinary Care

An illustration of the approach can be shown through the presentation of an 84-year-old patient. This patient had a low rectal tumor who had presented with symptomatic anemia and diarrhea with some incontinence. She had a background of hypertension and an adrenal lesion of unknown function at the point of diagnosis. Her daughter had left her and she brought up her granddaughter single-handedly. At the time of diagnosis, she was staying alone and cherished her independence despite her age and was keen not to have her cancer rob her of her independence. Treatment goals included curative resection with anal sphincter preservation and a rapid return to independence. Ultralow anterior resection with a temporary ileostomy was performed with discharge on the 8th postoperative day. The perioperative approach of the team is shown in Table 8.1. She subsequently underwent ileostomy closure uneventfully and had since been independent and continent. She had come to know the team involved in her management well and pays the team regular social visits. The team also visits her to ensure continued functional independence and social integration after the cancer treatment (Figs. 8.4 and 8.5).

Conclusion
There is no doubt that complex elderly patients will benefit from a holistic approach; however, achieving this requires high-level communication and coordination. Multidisciplinary care should make way for transdisciplinary care for these patients.

References

Caramanica L, Anderson R (2001) Transdisciplinary teams: lessons learned. Semin Nurse Manag 9(2):77–78
Christmas C, Makary MA et al (2006) Medical considerations in older surgical patients. J Am Coll Surg 203(5):746–751
Emmons KM, Viswanath K et al (2008) The role of transdisciplinary collaboration in translating and disseminating health research: lessons learned and exemplars of success. Am J Prev Med 35(2 Suppl):S204–S210
Mitchell PH (2005) What's in a name? Multidisciplinary, interdisciplinary, and transdisciplinary. J Prof Nurs 21(6):332–334
Reilly C (2001) Transdisciplinary approach: an atypical strategy for improving outcomes in rehabilitative and long-term acute care settings. Rehabil Nurs 26(6):216–220, 244
Walker LO, Avant KC (eds) (1995) Strategies for theory construction in nursing. Appleton & Lange, Norwalk
Wilson PR (1996) Multidisciplinary… transdisciplinary… monodisciplinary… where are we going? Clin J Pain 12(4):253–254

Anesthesia and Intraoperative Care of Elderly Surgery Patients

9

Edwin Seet and Frances Chung

Take Home Pearls

- Informed consent from the geriatric surgical patient may pose challenges due to sensory deficits and cognitive impairment.
- Optimization of preexisting disease in the elderly is important in improving outcomes. Careful medication reconciliation should be performed especially when there is polypharmacy.
- Intraoperative anesthesia care focuses on airway management, judicious fluid management, meticulous thermoregulation, use of short-acting anesthetic agents, multimodal analgesia, and regional techniques.
- Postoperative management involves a team-based interdisciplinary management approach with emphasis on pain management and ameliorating the adverse effects of postoperative cognitive dysfunction cum delirium.

E. Seet, MBBS MMed (✉)
Department of Anesthesia, Alexandra Health Private
Limited, Khoo Teck Puat Hospital,
90 Yishun Central, 768828 Singapore, Singapore
e-mail: seetedwin@gmail.com

F. Chung, MBBS FRCPC
Department of Anesthesia, University Health Network, University of Toronto,
399 Bathurst Street McL 2-405, Toronto, ON M5T 2S8, Canada
e-mail: frances.chung@uhn.ca

K.-Y. Tan (ed.), *Colorectal Cancer in the Elderly*,
DOI 10.1007/978-3-642-29883-7_9, © Springer-Verlag Berlin Heidelberg 2013

9.1   Introduction

The healthcare industry faces an acceleration of population aging (Lutz et al. 2008). The practice of anesthesiologists will progressively consist of more elderly patients as population longevity increases in tandem with the need for surgical intervention. The concept of the elderly or geriatric patient is best understood in terms of their functional status and comorbidities rather than merely a function of chronological age. These elderly patients pose particular healthcare challenges in the perioperative period (Silverstein 2009).

Poignant issues of geriatric anesthesia would include the nuances in obtaining informed consent, optimization of multiple complex coexisting disease, management of polypharmacy, intraoperative anesthesia care, and postoperative prevention of complications and continuity of care. Meticulous management of the elderly surgical patient is of paramount importance as they take significantly longer to return to their preoperative state and often never return to their baseline functional status (Lawrence et al. 2004).

9.2   Pre-anesthesia Considerations

9.2.1   Informed Consent

Informed consent may be defined as the process of communication between the medical professional and the patient in such a manner that the patient has a clear appreciation and understanding of the facts, the implications, and the consequences of the proposed surgery. This is particularly challenging for the elderly patient because of barriers to this communication process. Such barriers would include sensory deficits, cognitive impairment, hearing impairment, visual loss, and dementia. End of life discussions and intensive care unit admissions should also be discussed with the elderly patient prior to surgery. Often, family members or other surrogate decision makers may have to be engaged in the preoperative communication process.

9.2.2   Comorbidities

A general physical decline of multiple systems and a high prevalence of chronic disease accompany aging. Providing anesthesia for the elderly can be a particularly complex task, especially with the interplay of multiple patient comorbidities. In fact, a recent American study found an increased risk of anesthesia-related mortality in patients with advancing age (Li et al. 2009). The prevalence of preexisting medical diseases increases with increasing age. These medical comorbidities influence the risk of anesthesia and surgery. A list of such medical conditions includes but not limited to hypertension, atrial fibrillation, congestive heart failure, aortic valve sclerosis, diastolic dysfunction, obstructive sleep apnea, diabetes mellitus, hypothyroidism, Parkinson's disease, cerebrovascular disease, and renal impairment.

Preoperative risk assessment and optimization of these comorbidities would be important in mitigating the risk of perioperative morbidity in the geriatric patient. Judicious continuation of chronic medications should be done to ameliorate patient risk factors from comorbidities. Perioperative beta blockers have been shown to be protective against myocardial infarction, but increase the risk of stroke and total mortality. These risks were noted with higher doses of metoprolol (100 mg) which may result in severe bradycardia and hypotension (Devereaux et al. 2008). Perioperative statins, aspirin, and alpha 2 agonists may be useful in decreasing cardiovascular events, and these agents are the subject of current and future research. Occasionally, subspecialty referrals to the cardiologist, pulmonologist, endocrinologist, or geriatrician may be necessary to address complex patient-specific medical comorbidities.

9.2.3 Polypharmacy

As a result of the multiple comorbidities, elderly patients may be on a number of different medications. In fact, from a recent survey, it was reported that more than 90% of patients older than 65 years of age use at least one drug per week, 40% take five or more drugs, and 12–19% use 10 or more medications (Barnett 2009). Polypharmacy will result in difficulty with perioperative medication reconciliation. Furthermore, there may be potential interactions with drugs used in anesthesia, for example, anti-Parkinson drugs and opioids causing muscle rigidity (Nicholson et al. 2002). A team-based perioperative care of the elderly surgical patient including the expertise of a clinical pharmacist and geriatrician may be considered in the provision of optimal patient care.

9.2.4 Suitability for Ambulatory Surgery

The anesthesiologist is posed with a dilemma in the decision of whether surgery for a geriatric patient should be performed on an ambulatory basis. Consideration in favor of ambulatory surgery would include less disruption in lifestyle and the familiar home environment, reduced risk of hospital infections for the compromised elderly immune system, and a lesser loss of autonomy. In addition, there is some evidence that outpatient surgeries are associated with reduced risk of postoperative cognitive disorders (Canet et al. 2003). On the other side of the scale, these potential advantages of ambulatory surgery for the elderly patient have to be balanced against caregiver availability, basal medical conditions, and patient-cum-family comprehension (Bettelli 2010; Bryson et al. 2004).

9.3 Intraoperative Anesthetic Care

9.3.1 Airway Assessment

The airway is often the quintessential concern for the anesthesiologist. Older patients are sometime edentulous; they have vulnerable irregular dentition and limited neck mobility. The combination of these factors may result in the geriatric airway being difficult to manage, both in terms of mask ventilation and tracheal intubation with direct laryngoscopy. A heightened index of suspicion and adequate preoperative airway assessment would help the anesthesiologists identify the potentially difficult airway, so that preparations may be made in anticipation of the difficult airway. Video laryngoscopes and other airway adjuncts may be made available prior to the induction of anesthesia.

9.3.2 Thermoregulation

Hypothermia is associated with adverse postoperative outcomes including increased incidence of blood loss, wound infection, and even in-hospital mortality (Karalapillai et al. 2009). Elderly patient is particularly susceptible because of age-related diminution of thermoregulatory control. Vigilance in core temperature monitoring and meticulous intervention to prevent heat loss by the anesthesiologist would prove to be important in improving outcomes for the geriatric population. Various methods of perioperative patient warming are known and commonly available; unfortunately they remain underutilized. Prewarming patients prior to the induction of anesthesia reduces hypothermia arising from heat redistribution. Intraoperative use of forced-air warming, heating intravenous fluids, and circulating water garments also have been shown to be effective maintaining normothermia.

9.3.3 Fluid Regimen and Blood Transfusion Triggers

The issue of what type of fluids, how much to administer, and when to transfuse blood products have been controversial topics of research and academic argument in recent years. Crystalloids versus colloids, restrictive versus liberal fluid therapy, and restrictive versus liberal transfusion approaches have been debated vigorously. Unfortunately, an unambiguous solution has not been found because of lack of consensus, as well as heterogeneity in research methodology of existing studies (Bundgaard-Nielsen et al. 2009). Crystalloid overload, hyperchloremic acidosis from 0.9% sodium chloride, and overtransfusion of stored blood may result in adverse outcomes and should be avoided. On the other hand, judicious time-oriented goal-directed patient-specific fluid management strategies to maintain normovolemia and concurrent prevention of blood loss may ameliorate perioperative insults from surgery and anesthesia.

9.3.4   Anesthesia in the Elderly

The use of anesthetic agents in the geriatric patient must be adjusted and titrated according to response because of altered pharmacokinetic and pharmacodynamic changes in the elderly. Opioids, inhalational agents, intravenous induction agents, and muscle relaxants all have an impact on the elderly patient's cardio-cerebro-pulmonary physiology, leading to undesired hemodynamic depression, respiratory compromise, and delayed recovery. Drug dosages may be reduced by up to 20–50% in the elderly. Attentive monitoring and feedback of these vital systems should be routinely considered with the use of end-tidal anesthetic gas monitors, brain function monitors (e.g., processed electroencephalography), train-of-four neuromuscular stimulators, target control infusion pumps (Schnider model), and perhaps even closed loop propofol administration systems.

Emergence from anesthesia may be particularly challenging in the elderly patient. Reasons for delayed awakening may be the result of multifactorial interactions between medical comorbidities, pathophysiological processes of aging, and anesthetic agents administered. The anesthesiologist has to be cognizant of the differential diagnoses of delayed awakening and the principles of managing these pharmacological, biochemical, metabolic and neurologic etiologies, so that appropriate investigations cum interventions may be performed (Anastasian et al. 2009).

9.3.5   Regional Anesthesia and Perioperative Analgesia

Optimal pain management can ameliorate major postoperative complications (Liu and Wu 2007). Continuous or single-shot regional techniques with local anesthetics (alone or in combination with general anesthesia), local anesthesia infiltration, and opioid-sparing multimodal analgesia techniques may help to mitigate the deleterious effects of intravenous opioids and anesthetics in the vulnerable elderly patient.

9.4   Postoperative Continuity of Care

9.4.1   Postoperative Delirium and Cognitive Dysfunction

Postoperative cognitive dysfunction and postoperative delirium are common complications in the elderly with reported incidences in the range of 40% and 25%, respectively. Unfortunately, these conditions are often undiagnosed and under-appreciated by healthcare providers, despite evidence that both these conditions are associated with higher morbidity and even mortality rates (Steinmetz et al. 2009).

Postoperative delirium is characterized by a fluctuating change in cognition with a severe disturbance in attention and thinking, and an affected level of consciousness. Unmodifiable risk factors are age and preexisting dementia. Other risk factors include drugs, dehydration, sensory deprivation, and anxiety (Robinson et al. 2009). Treatment of postoperative delirium is focused on the prevention of modifiable precipitating factors. The anesthesiologist may be able to optimize glucose control, electrolytes, and hemoglobin levels; minimize the use of long-acting benzodiazepines; and manage postoperative pain (Sieber 2009). Therapeutic medication for postoperative delirium should involve the collaborative input from the geriatrician.

In contrast, postoperative cognitive dysfunction does not result in alteration in the level of consciousness and usually involves a more persistent decline in the elderly patient's functionality – memory, concentration, and information processing (Ramaiah and Lam 2009). It is a neurocognitive disorder characteristically associated with a decline in the performance of activities of daily living in the elderly patient. Etiological factors include age, educational level, duration of anesthesia, and multiple operations.

An interdisciplinary team-based approach involving key clinicians (surgeons, anesthesiologists, geriatricians, clinical pharmacists, dieticians, physiotherapists) will be needed to help mitigate the adverse effects of both postoperative delirium and cognitive dysfunction. Management strategies in the postoperative period would include early enteral nutrition, good analgesia regimes, early mobilization, and emotional support.

9.4.2 Pain Management

Anesthesiologists are confronted with difficulties in postoperative pain management in the elderly patient. In the face of possible hearing and visual impairment, cognitive disturbances, dementia, aphasia, and lack of comprehension of pain scales, observational pain assessment tools may have to be utilized. Postoperative multimodal analgesia techniques are useful and aim to reduce adverse effects of single analgesic modalities such as respiratory depression and confusion from opioids, as well as gastric and renal impairment from nonsteroidal anti-inflammatory drugs.

Conclusion

The geriatric patient with multiple comorbidities requiring anesthesia for major surgery will constitute a substantial proportion of the anesthesiologist's practice in the years to come.

Future opportunities in the field of geriatric anesthesia should focus professional education of evidence-based guidelines on the optimization and management of geriatric patient-specific comorbidities (Deiner and Silverstein 2011), research in ameliorating perioperative complications such as postoperative cognitive dysfunction and delirium, and the provision of perioperative continuity of care by interdisciplinary clinical team.

References

Anastasian ZH, Ornstein E, Heyer EJ (2009) Delayed arousal. Anesthesiol Clin 27:429–450

Barnett SR (2009) Polypharmacy and perioperative medications in the elderly. Anesthesiol Clin 27:377–389

Bettelli G (2010) Anaesthesia for the elderly outpatient: preoperative assessment and evaluation, anaesthetic technique and postoperative pain management. Curr Opin Anaesthesiol 23:726–731

Bryson GL, Chung F, Finegan BA, Friedman Z, Miller DR, van Vlymen J, Cox RG, Crowe MJ, Fuller J, Henderson C (2004) Patient selection in ambulatory anesthesia – an evidence-based review: part I. Can J Anaesth 51:768–781

Bundgaard-Nielsen M, Secher NH, Kehlet H (2009) "Liberal" vs. "restrictive" perioperative fluid therapy – a critical assessment of the evidence. Acta Anaesthesiol Scand 53:843–851

Canet J, Raeser J, Rasmussen LS et al (2003) Cognitive dysfunction after minor surgery in the elderly. Acta Anaesthesiol Scand 47:1204–1210

Deiner S, Silverstein JH (2011) Anesthesia for geriatric patients. Minerva Anestesiol 77:180–189

Devereaux PJ, Yang H, Yusuf S, Guyatt G, Leslier K et al (2008) Effects of extended-release metoprolol succinate in patients undergoing non-cardiac surgery (POISE trial): a randomised controlled trial. Lancet 371:1839–1847

Karalapillai D, Story DA, Calzavacca P, Licari E, Liu YL, Hart GK (2009) Inadvertent hypothermia and mortality in postoperative intensive care patients: retrospective audit of 5050 patients. Anaesthesia 64:968–972

Lawrence VA, Hazuda HP, Cornell JE, Pederson T, Bradshaw PT, Mulrow CD et al (2004) Functional independence after major abdominal surgery in the elderly. J Am Coll Surg 199:762–772

Li G, Warner M, Lang BH, Huang L, Sun LS (2009) Epidemiology of anesthesia-related mortality in the United States 1999–2005. Anesthesiology 110:759–765

Liu SS, Wu CL (2007) Effect of postoperative analgesia on major postoperative complications: a systematic update of the evidence. Anesth Analg 104:689–702

Lutz W, Sanderson W, Scherbov S (2008) The coming acceleration of global population ageing. Nature 451:716–719

Nicholson G, Pereira AC, Hall GM (2002) Parkinson's disease and anaesthesia. Br J Anaesth 89:904–916

Ramaiah R, Lam AM (2009) Postoperative cognitive dysfunction in the elderly. Anesthesiol Clin 27:485–496

Robinson TN, Raeburn CD, Tran ZV, Angles EM, Brenner LA, Moss M (2009) Postoperative delirium in the elderly: risk factors and outcomes. Ann Surg 249:173–178

Sieber FE (2009) Postoperative delirium in the elderly surgical patient. Anesthesiol Clin 27:451–464

Silverstein J (2009) Problems with geriatric anesthesia patients. Anesthesiol Clin 27:xv–xvi

Steinmetz J, Christensen KB, Lund T, Lohse N, Rasmussen LS, ISPOCD Group (2009) Long-term consequences of postoperative cognitive dysfunction. Anesthesiology 110:548–555

Minimally Invasive Surgery for Colorectal Cancer in the Elderly Patients

10

Fumio Konishi

Take Home Pearls

- Because of the less invasive nature of laparoscopic colectomy, it is a good indication for elderly patients with colorectal diseases.
- Provided the surgical risk factors in the elderly patients are evaluated carefully, laparoscopic surgery will result in a good short-term as well as long-term outcome for colorectal cancer patients.

10.1 Introduction

There is an increasing population of elderly people in Western as well as in Asian countries. According to the government statistics of Japan, in the year 2010, the population of people older than 64 years of age had reached 29 million, which was 23.1% of the total population in Japan. It is expected that in the year 2015, the population of people older than 64 will reach 30 million which is 30.5% of the total population. The percentage of elderly people in Japan is the highest in the world. As the population of the older people increases, the surgeons are operating on more and more elderly patients. Because of the increasing tendency of the elderly patients, 60–70 years of age is not considered old. The rate of comorbidity in the elderly patients is higher and also frailty is more often present in the elderly

F. Konishi
Department of Surgery, Nerima Hikarigaoka Hospital,
Tokyo, Japan
e-mail: DZD00740@nifty.ne.jp

K.-Y. Tan (ed.), *Colorectal Cancer in the Elderly*,
DOI 10.1007/978-3-642-29883-7_10, © Springer-Verlag Berlin Heidelberg 2013

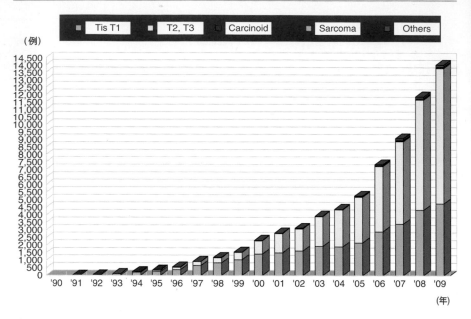

Fig. 10.1 Nationwide statistics of laparoscopic colorectal surgery in Japan (Journal of Japan Society of Endoscpoic Surgery (2010))

patients. Therefore, the surgical intervention and operative risks should carefully be evaluated during perioperative period when elderly patients need to receive surgical operations.

In the elderly patients, there is an increasing incidence of malignant tumors of the digestive organs, prostate in males, lung, and other organs. Among these malignant tumors, colorectal cancer is one of the most frequently seen tumors in the elderly. In elderly patients as well as in younger patients, many of the colorectal cancers can be curable if surgical resection is safely carried out.

Since the first report by Jacobs in 1991 (Jacobs et al. 1991), laparoscopic colorectal surgery has been practiced with an increasing number of cases each year. Most of the cases of laparoscopic colorectal surgery in Japan are cancer cases. According the nationwide statistics in Japan, in the year 2009, fourteen hundred cases of laparoscopic colorectal cancer surgery were performed (JSES 2010) (Fig. 10.1). According to the statistics of reimbursement of medical insurance, the take-up rate of laparoscopic colon cancer surgery was approximately 30% in 2009. The take-up rate will rise due to the recognition of superiority of the procedure over open surgery and also due to the wider availability of the technique (Fig. 10.2).

As laparoscopic colorectal surgery is less invasive than open surgery, it will be a good indication for elderly patients who tend to have comorbidity and/or frailty. However, in laparoscopic colorectal surgery, there are such problems as longer operation time and the adverse effects due to the pneumoperitoneum. Therefore, it is mandatory to analyze whether laparoscopic colorectal surgery is safe and truly beneficial to elderly patients in short-term as well as in long-term.

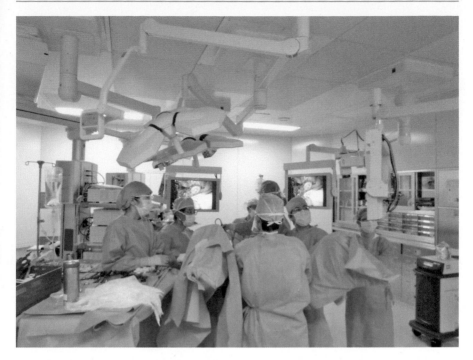

Fig. 10.2 Laparoscopic colectomy, setting of the operating room

10.2   Definition of Elderly Patients in Colorectal Cancer Patients

Because patients with colorectal diseases, particularly colorectal cancer, are becoming older and older, it seems that according to our experience, patients 65–75 years old are not generally considered as "old" (Tan et al. 2010). In the reported studies on laparoscopic colorectal surgery, the age of the elderly patients differ. There are four studies in which octogenarians who underwent laparoscopic colectomy were studied (Vignali et al. 2005; Stewart et al. 1999; Cheung et al. 2007; Issa et al. 2011). In other studies, the defined ages were 65, 70, or 75. In Japan, the ministry of health defined the age of the elderly as 65 or older. The elderly people are further divided into two. The patients between 65 and 74 are defined as "young old," and those 75 or over are defined as "old old." Therefore, in Japan in our clinical study, it seems that the patients 75 or older will be the appropriate definition of elderly patients (Tan and Konishi 2010). In UK, colorectal cancer collaborative group reported that patients between 65 and 70 should not be considered old from a physiological and functional point of view.

10.3   Surgical Risks and Their Evaluation

To evaluate the surgical risk, there are several commonly used assessment tools. The predictive factors of postoperative morbidity and mortality are mostly based on the retrospective analysis of patients who underwent surgery with known outcomes.

Various factors including symptoms, comorbidities, and laboratory data have been
identified as important surgical risk factors. The age itself may not be a risk factor,
but comorbidities and frailty associated with the old age are considered to be risk
factors of surgical patients.

There are several well-used scoring systems for the assessment of surgical risk
which has also been used for colorectal cancer patients. All of the scoring systems
are used for both elderly and non-elderly patients, but some of them are considered
particularly useful for the elderly patients.

10.3.1 American Society of Anesthesiologists ASA Scores

This is the most widely used scoring system (Bowles et al. 2008). The mortality rates
for Class I, II, IV, and V were reported as 0.08%, 1.8%, 7.8%, and 9.8%. Commonly,
the preoperative assessment of patients with Class II and III is important.

10.3.2 Physiological and Operative Severity Score
for the Enumeration of Mortality and Morbidity
(POSSUM, CR-POSSUM)

The efficacy of POSSUM for the prediction of the postoperative outcome has
been proven. This scoring system is widely used because of the relative simplicity
and proven efficacy. The parameters are age, respiratory and cardiac co-morbidities,
ECG, blood pressure, BUN, Hb WBC, electroplaters, grade of operative intervention, blood loss, malignant tumor, and intraperitoneal bacterial contamination.
With this scoring, postoperative morbidity and mortality rate will be automati-
cally analyzed. However, there is a tendency to overestimate the operative risk of
elderly patient with this scoring system. CR-POSSUM is subsequently developed
using multivariate models of colorectal surgery and based on the same principles
(Horzic et al. 2007). This model also may overestimate the surgical risk of elderly
patients.

10.3.3 Charlson Weighted Comorbidity Index

This index is more commonly used by geriatricians. This index gives each comorbidity a different weight according to the long-term outcome of patients with particular comorbidities. This index gives each comorbidity a different weight and is
helpful in quantifying the comorbidities in the elderly patients (Charlson et al.
1987). Our recent study on colorectal surgery patients showed that the risk of post-
operative comorbidity was almost four times higher if the weighted comorbidity
index core was 5 or greater (Tan et al. 2009).

10.3.4 Frailty

"Frailty" is a new concept in assessing the surgical risk of elderly patients. It is interesting to note that some of the elderly patients without comorbidity may show higher frailty index. The presence of frailty is determined based on the activity level, grip strength, and walking speed as suggested by Fried et al. (2001).

10.4   General Aspects of the Reports on Laparoscopic Colectomy in the Elderly Patients

There are a number of studies on laparoscopic colorectal surgery in the elderly. However, the nature of these studies is retrospective, and randomized controlled trials have not been reported. The main problem of the retrospective nature of the previous studies is the possible selection bias of patients for laparoscopic surgery in the elderly. It is controversial whether laparoscopic colorectal surgery, which usually takes a longer time and also has an increased risk of CO_2 accumulation due to pneumoperitoneum, can be indicated for patients with moderate to severe cardiopulmonary complications. It seems that elderly patients with severe cardiopulmonary diseases tended to be excluded from the laparoscopic surgery and to receive open surgery. In most of the previous reports on laparoscopic colectomy in the elderly patients, the indication of this procedure with comorbidities was not well stated. Because randomized controlled trials comparing laparoscopic vs open in elderly patients with comorbidities is extremely difficult to perform, we need to analyze and discuss the outcome of laparoscopic colorectal surgery for the elderly patients based on the retrospective data analyses.

10.5   Comparison Between Laparoscopic Colorectal Cancer Surgery and Open Surgery in the Elderly

10.5.1 Comparison Between Laparoscopic Versus Open Surgery in the Elderly

There are three reports on octogenarians (Cheung et al. 2007; Stewart et al. 1999; Vignali et al. 2005; Issa et al. 2011). In these reports, laparoscopic colectomy for cancer was compared to open colectomy; the authors discussed that although the operation time was longer in laparoscopic surgery, the length of the hospital stay was shorter in LC and postoperative complication rate tended to be lower in laparoscopic surgery. Vignali reported in their case-matched study that the worsening of the independence score was significantly less in laparoscopic surgery than in open surgery advocating less invasive nature of laparoscopic surgery (Vignali et al. 2005). However, in these reports, it was not clearly stated how the patients were selected for laparoscopic procedure. Cheung analyzed 101 octogenarian patients who underwent laparoscopic colorectal cancer surgery and reported that median operation time was 110 min, blood loss was 50, conversion occurred in only one patient, and postoperative morbidity and mortality rates were 17% and 3%. They concluded that laparoscopic colectomy for octogenarian is safe and carries better short-term results (Cheung et al. 2007). Their selection criteria for laparoscopic surgery were those fit for surgical treatment, without multiple abdominal operations, without locally advanced tumors. Therefore, it is considered that in their practice, there are no special indications for laparoscopic colorectal surgery in the elderly that are different from those for open surgery.

Other short-term postoperative studies comparing laparoscopic vs open in elderly patients (age 70 or older/75 or older) also demonstrated the advantages of laparoscopic colectomy over open colectomy (Delgado et al. 2000; Law et al. 2002; Tei et al. 2009). The results of these reports demonstrated that although the length of operation was longer in laparoscopic colectomy, the postoperative hospital stay was shorter and the return of bowel function was earlier. Law reported that comparing laparoscopic colectomy vs open colectomy in patients 70 or older, the two groups did not show differences in ASA score and yet there was a significantly lower postoperative cardiopulmonary complication in the laparoscopic colectomy patients than in open cases (Law et al. 2002). Including the report by Wai et al., in most of the studies, the selection criteria for laparoscopic colorectal cancer surgery for elderly patients were not clearly documented. It is of interest to note that in the study reported by Tei et al. prognostic nutritional index of open colectomy patients was significantly lower than that of laparoscopic colectomy patients, which may suggest that that laparoscopic colectomy might have been selected for patients with better nutritional status comparing to the open surgery patients. In their report, the postoperative complication rate was lower in laparoscopic than in open surgery patients which might well be due to the better nutritional status of the patients who underwent laparoscopic colectomy (Tei et al. 2009).

10.5.2 Comparison with Younger Patients

There are several studies in which laparoscopic colectomy were compared between elderly and younger patients. In our own study reported by Tan et al., 91 laparoscopic colorectal cancer surgery patients who were 75 years or older were compared with 379 laparoscopic colorectal cancer surgery patients under 70 years of age. There was no difference in the occurrence of postoperative complications between the two groups. Multivariate analysis revealed that patient's age was not an independent risk factor of major complications. There were 4 deaths within 30 postoperative day. Although bivariate analysis revealed that older age was a significant risk factor for mortality, multivariate analysis showed that Charlson comorbidity index and operation time but not age were independent

Table 10.1 Multivariate analysis for risk factors for major complications

Factor	Odds ratio	95% CI	P
Male sex	2.0	1.0–3.8	0.044
Rectal surgery	2.4	1.1–5.5	0.032
Cardiac disease	2.6	0.9–7.0	0.062
Previous cerebrovascular accident	2.7	0.5–14.0	0.230
Comorbidity index ≥5	1.1	0.1–60.6	0.604
Conversion	1.0	0.4–2.9	0.881
Blood loss			0.044
Operative time			0.353
Mean comorbidity index score			0.137

Tan et al. (2010)

Table 10.2 Multivariate analysis for risk factors of 30-day mortality

Factor	Odds ratio	95% CI	P
Age ≥75	15.8	0.4–669.6	0.149
Cardiac disease	0.2	0.1–31.5	0.541
Previous cerebrovascular accident	3.8	0.1–489.1	0.587
Comorbidity index ≥5	1557.4	4.2–584,085	0.015
Operative time			0.012

Tan et al. (2010)

risk factors for mortality, and we concluded that laparoscopic colorectal surgery should not be denied based on age alone (Tan et al. 2010) (Tables 10.1 and 10.2). Other studies also showed no significant differences in postoperative morbidity between elderly and younger patients (Senagore et al. 2003; Sklow et al. 2003; Person et al. 2008).

Fiscon et al. also reported a comparative study on postoperative complications of laparoscopic colectomy between elderly and younger patients (Fiscon et al. 2010). This report is of importance because 95.6% of 226 patients in their series that include both elderly and younger patients underwent laparoscopic colectomy. Therefore, the bias for choosing laparoscopic colectomy in both elderly and in younger patients is considered to be minimal. Their results showed that although postoperative surgical complications were similar in elderly and younger patients, the postoperative medical complications were significantly higher in the elderly patients. This results presented higher vulnerability in the elderly patients than in younger patients when laparoscopic colorectal cancer surgery was performed. They also discussed that these results may well be due to the higher ASA score in the elderly patients (Table 10.3). The authors further stated that age per se should not be considered a contraindication to laparoscopic colorectal surgery.

Table 10.3 Postoperative complications (total $n=216$)

Complication	<75 years old ($n=134$)	75 years old and above ($n=82$)	P
Surgical	8 (5.9)	7 (8.5)	0.58
Anastomotic leak	3 (2.2)	1 (1.2)	
Volvulus	0	1 (1.2)	
Enterocutaneous fistula	0	1 (1.2)	
Abdominal collection	1 (0.7)	0	
Hemorrhage	0	0	
Wound infection	2 (1.5)	4 (4.9)	
Other	12 (1.5)	0	
Medical	5 (3.7)	12 (14.5)	0.007
Pneumonia	0	2 (2.4)	
Pulmonary embolism	1 (0.7)	0	
Deep venous thrombosis	0	1 (1.2)	
Atrial fibrillation	0	3 (3.6)	
Renal failure	0	1 (1.2)	
Other	4 (3)	5 (6.1)	
Total	13 (9.7)	19 (23.2)	0.01
Reoperations	1 (0.7)	2 (2.4)	0.56

Fiscon et al. (2010)

10.6 Long-Term Oncological Outcomes in the Elderly Patients Who Underwent Laparoscopic Surgery

Although there are a number of reports on the oncological outcomes of laparoscopic colorectal cancer surgery including several randomized controlled studies (Fleshman et al. 2007; Kitano et al. 2005; Lacy et al. 2008). There are only a few reports on the long-term outcome of colorectal laparoscopic cancer surgery in the elderly patients Nakamura et al. analyzed ontological outcome of laparoscopy surgery in the elderly patients with colon cancer (Nakamura et al. 2011). They compared 74 patients who were 75 years or older and 74 patients who were 64 years or younger, and concluded that long-term oncological outcomes were similar in elderly patients and younger painters with colon cancer who underwent laparoscopic colectomy. However, the number of patients they studied was limited and large-scale study on the oncological outcome in the elderly patients who underwent laparoscopic colorectal cancer surgery should be analyzed in the future.

Conclusions

Most of the retrospective studies showed that laparoscopic colorectal surgery in the elderly patients can safely be performed as in the younger patients. However, due to the retrospective nature of the studies, still it is not clearly determined whether elderly patients with comorbidities can safely be operated on as in younger patients with similar comorbidities. As the indication for laparoscopic colectomy in the elderly patients expands including those with high-grade cardiopulmonary comorbidities, it should be further investigated whether the indication for laparoscopic colectomy can similarly be indicated in the elderly as in the younger patients.

References

Bowles TA, Sanders KM et al (2008) Simplified risk stratification in elective colorectal surgery. ANZ J Surg 78(1–2):24–27

Charlson ME, Pompei P et al (1987) A new method of classifying prognostic comorbidity in longitudinal studies: development and validation. J Chronic Dis 40(5):373–383

Cheung HY, Chung CC et al (2007) Laparoscopic resection for colorectal cancer in octogenarians: results in a decade. Dis Colon Rectum 50(11):1905–1910

Delgado S, Lacy AM et al (2000) Could age be an indication for laparoscopic colectomy in colorectal cancer? Surg Endosc 14(1):22–26

Fiscon V, Portale G et al (2010) Laparoscopic resection of colorectal cancer in elderly patients. Tumori 96(5):704–708

Fleshman J, Sargent DJ et al (2007) Laparoscopic colectomy for cancer is not inferior to open surgery based on 5-year data from the COST Study Group trial. Ann Surg 246(4):655–662; discussion 662–4

Fried LP, Tangen CM et al (2001) Frailty in older adults: evidence for a phenotype. J Gerontol A Biol Sci Med Sci 56(3):M146–M156

Horzic M, Kopljar M et al (2007) Comparison of P-POSSUM and Cr-POSSUM scores in patients undergoing colorectal cancer resection. Arch Surg 142(11):1043–1048

Issa N, Grassi C et al (2011) Laparoscopic colectomy for carcinoma of the colon in octogenarians. J Gastrointest Surg 15:2011–2015

Jacobs M, Verdeja JC et al (1991) Minimally invasive colon resection (laparoscopic colectomy). Surg Laparosc Endosc 1(3):144–150

JSES (2010) Nationwide statistics of laparoscopic surgery in Japan. J Jpn Soc Endosc Surg 15(5):565–671

Kitano S, Inomata M et al (2005) Randomized controlled trial to evaluate laparoscopic surgery for colorectal cancer: Japan Clinical Oncology Group Study JCOG 0404. Jpn J Clin Oncol 35(8):475–477

Lacy AM, Delgado S et al (2008) The long-term results of a randomized clinical trial of laparoscopy-assisted versus open surgery for colon cancer. Ann Surg 248(1):1–7

Law WL, Chu KW et al (2002) Laparoscopic colorectal resection: a safe option for elderly patients. J Am Coll Surg 195(6):768–773

Nakamura T, Mitomi H et al (2011) Oncological outcomes of laparoscopic surgery in elderly patients with colon cancer: a comparison of patients 64 years or younger with those 75 years or older. Hepatogastroenterology 58(109):1200–1204

Person B, Cera SM et al (2008) Do elderly patients benefit from laparoscopic colorectal surgery? Surg Endosc 22(2):401–405

Senagore AJ, Madbouly KM et al (2003) Advantages of laparoscopic colectomy in older patients. Arch Surg 138(3):252–256

Sklow B, Read T et al (2003) Age and type of procedure influence the choice of patients for laparoscopic colectomy. Surg Endosc 17(6):923–929

Stewart BT, Stitz RW et al (1999) Laparoscopically assisted colorectal surgery in the elderly. Br J Surg 86(7):938–941

Tan KY, Kawamura Y et al (2009) Colorectal surgery in octogenarian patients – outcomes and predictors of morbidity. Int J Colorectal Dis 24(2):185–189

Tan KY, Konishi F (2010) Long-term results of laparoscopic colorectal cancer resection: current knowledge and what remains unclear. Surg Today 40(2):97–101

Tan KY, Konishi F et al (2010) Laparoscopic colorectal surgery in elderly patients: a case-control study of 15 years of experience. Am J Surg 201(4):531–536

Tei M, Ikeda M et al (2009) Postoperative complications in elderly patients with colorectal cancer: comparison of open and laparoscopic surgical procedures. Surg Laparosc Endosc Percutan Tech 19(6):488–492

Vignali A, Di Palo S et al (2005) Laparoscopic vs. open colectomies in octogenarians: a case-matched control study. Dis Colon Rectum 48(11):2070–2075

Truths and Myths of Postoperative Care for the Elderly

11

William J. Speake

Take Home Pearls

- Elderly patients are high-risk patients and are more at risk of general as opposed to surgical site complications.
- Delirium is frequently encountered, may well be preventable and is often managed poorly.
- Whilst critical care is often essential in the early post-operative period, a holistic approach is needed; carers need to be aware of the risks of functional decline at all stages of postoperative recovery, including post-discharge.
- Enhanced recovery provides an excellent framework for the elderly patient's post-operative course and may need to be adapted but is entirely appropriate.
- Elderly patients are at particular risk of fluid miss-management, poor pain control and malnutrition.
- Standard adult guidelines may need to be adapted for the elderly patient.

11.1 Introduction

The post-operative care of an elderly colorectal surgery patient should be dictated by good preoperative assessment, and in all cases, they should be considered high risk. Elderly patients are frequently at increased risk of complication due to co-morbidity, and in turn increasing co-morbidity is associated with poorer outcome (Pedrazzani et al. 2009). Limited physiological reserves mean that complications are tolerated

W.J. Speake
Department of Surgery,
Derby Colorectal Unit, Royal Derby Hospital,
Derby DE22 3NE, UK
e-mail: william.speake@derbyhospitals.nhs.uk

K.-Y. Tan (ed.), *Colorectal Cancer in the Elderly*,
DOI 10.1007/978-3-642-29883-7_11, © Springer-Verlag Berlin Heidelberg 2013

poorly, and once they become established, an inevitable decline with grave consequences frequently follows. Critical care, subsequent observant step-down care, prior to returning elderly patients to a safe home or rehabilitation environment whilst continually preventing functional decline, is of paramount importance. Notwithstanding these points, this group of patients are still entirely suitable and will benefit immensely from enhanced recovery protocols. The aims of good post-operative care should be to detect and treat any complication at its earliest possible stage whilst rehabilitating the patient back to their optimal functional state. In practice, there are many misunderstood beliefs regarding elderly patients; in this chapter, we explore various myths and truths so that post-operative care for the elderly patient can be optimized.

11.2 Elderly Patients Have the Same Complications as Younger Patients but More Frequently

It cannot be argued that elderly patients have an equivalent frequency of overall complications to younger patients. A spectrum of typical complication rates is presented in Table 11.1. However, with closer scrutiny of the presented data, what we actually see is that specific complications are increased in the elderly population and particularly in the emergency setting. Overall major complications are almost doubled in Tan's study (mean age 85 (80–106)) for emergency procedures as compared to elective (Tan et al. 2006). This has also been borne out in other large series (Tan et al. 2007; Basili et al. 2008; CCCG 2000). This is an important consideration as elderly patients will often present late and are more likely to undergo emergency procedures. This data suggests that the argument that 'this elderly patient is high risk so we won't operate electively rather wait until they obstruct or develop another complication' is fundamentally flawed. If this approach is followed, thus pushing your patient into a high-risk emergency group, then you are in essence arguing that the patient should not be operated upon at all. Facing inevitable problems electively and early, if a patient is a surgical candidate, is a far better approach.

Another common misheld belief is that the elderly patient is at higher risk of anastomotic dehiscence with a resulting increase in stoma rates. Whilst the elderly patient may have limited physiological reserve to deal with any leak, examining the data demonstrates that leak rates are not increased in all the above studies. So which complications are the elderly most at risk of? Notably, there does not appear to be any greater risk of site-specific and local complications after surgery (e.g. bleeds, anastomotic dehiscence and wound complications). Conversely, the elderly are at more risk of general, and specifically, respiratory, cardiovascular and thromboembolic complications (CCCG 2000; Marusch et al. 2005; Tan et al. 2006). These 'general' complications need faultless prophylactic measures in the perioperative period to ensure good functional outcome; infective chest complications being the most frequent complication in elective groups and occurring even more often in the emergency setting. Furthermore,

Table 11.1 Complications following major abdominal surgery in octogenarians (%)

	Overall (n = 125)	Elective (n = 64)	Emergency (n = 61)
Acute coronary syndrome	9	6	12
Chest infection/atelectasis	30	22	38
Cerebrovascular event	2	3	2
Deep vein thrombosis	2	3	0
Acute renal failure	6	3	10
Wound infection	10	8	13
Anastomotic leak	2	2	3

Modified from Tan et al. (2006) with permission

post-operative delirium is a complication that occurs almost exclusively in the elderly and can occur in up to 50% of elderly patients. It is often managed poorly and associated with delayed recovery and poorer outcomes (Christmas et al. 2006). Aspiration, falls, dislodged tubes and wound problems are frequently associated once it occurs.

In essence, complications are increased; however, it seems to only be general as opposed to local complications.

11.3   Delirium Is a Frequent and Inevitable Complication in the Elderly Patient

Whilst delirium is a frequent occurrence, there are many preventative measures that can be put in place to either prevent it altogether or lessen its degree. Patient orientation is vital, rooms without windows should be avoided, and patients' own spectacles and hearing aids should be used as soon as possible after surgery. Ward changes should be limited to critical care to standard ward only. Friend and family visits, familiar faces, should be welcomed.

Other risk factors such as alcohol withdrawal, polypharmacy and poor nutrition should be considered and treated accordingly. Medication should be reviewed, not only that which the patient claims they are on, but have there been any recent additions, discontinuations or omissions? For example, a patient who has dementia may not have had their donepizil prescribed. Risk factors such as uncontrolled post-operative pain, hypoxia and unrecognized infections, particularly urinary tract infections, should be assessed and treated.

Dementia specialist nurses and geriatric physicians have a crucial role to play in prevention and management of post-operative delirium. On occasion, it may be necessary to resort to pharmacological treatment, but this should only be after a careful assessment of the situation and after the above measures have failed. Titration of antipsychotic drugs such as risperidone and haloperidol can be of use ideally in consultation with geriatric physicians (Tan et al. 2010; Halter et al. 2009). Delirium therefore is not inevitable, can often be lessened in degree if it does occur and can often be treated effectively in a multidisciplinary manner.

11.4 Monitoring Aggressively for Complications Is the Single Most Important Feature in Post-operative Care for the Elderly Patient

There is good evidence that a period of 2–3 days in critical care after major surgery is of great benefit (Cavaliere et al. 2008). This is predominantly to allow full recovery from a major anaesthetic but also to allow prompt recognition and treatment of any complication. Many hospitals do not have this facility in abundance and 'step down' to a normal ward with early warning scores and critical care outreach teams in place is another option. However, what we have to remember is that whilst we can become very much focussed on the specific post-operative recovery, we also have to pay heed to the functional recovery of the elderly patient. There is little point in returning an elderly patient to a previous home environment with a perfectly functioning stoma only for him to be unable to cope in that setting. A main 'raison d'être' of the senior surgeon coordinating the elderly patient care is to be perceptive for any evidence of functional decline. This has to flow through all post-operative periods from awakening from the anaesthetic to long beyond discharge home.

Many elderly patients may choose not to undergo major surgery if they are likely to lose their independence. Whilst many poor functional outcomes are seen as a result of post-operative morbidity, functional decline can and often does occur in its absence.

'Health is a state of complete physical, mental and social well being not merely the absence of disease. Life is not merely the absence of disease but to be well' (Chee and Tan 2010). If a patient does not return to a good quality of life following surgery, then that must be considered an error in patient selection or of functional rehabilitation, a patient who is left bed bound and was previously independent has had a failure in this pathway.

11.5 Post-operative Rehabilitation Has to Be at a Slower Pace than Younger Patients

There is good evidence the enhanced recovery multifaceted approach to perioperative care is extremely beneficial (Fig. 11.1) (Gouvas et al. 2009; Varadhan et al. 2010a, b). Often elderly patients do not benefit from enhanced recovery as it is felt to be inappropriate and more traditional post-operative regimens are followed. This is in fact a misinterpretation of the evidence; a lot of the principles can be followed, and in fact, the elderly can often benefit more. Giving a target discharge date will focus a patient's mind, limiting preoperative 'nil by mouth' periods and early reintroduction of fluids and diet will clearly be of benefit to a group of patients that are at risk from malnutrition. Early reintroduction of fluids is usually well tolerated and will limit the need for additional parenteral fluid therapy which often leads to gut oedema and ileus (Lobo et al. 2002).

Fig. 11.1 Factors involved in enhanced recovery protocols

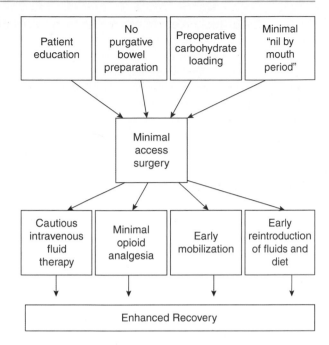

As we have discussed above, infective chest complications are by far the most frequent problem in the post-laparotomy elderly patient (Tan et al. 2006; CCCG 2000). Preoperative patient education on effective breathing techniques is widely held to be good practise (Doyle 1999) and is a component part of enhanced recovery. Early and aggressive chest physiotherapy, in tandem with good post-operative analgesia, is of paramount importance in getting a potentially frail and weak elderly patient to expectorate adequately. To this end, humidified oxygen and saline nebulisers are ideal. Respiratory reserve and chest compliance are frequently reduced in the elderly; hence, any progression of atelectasis to frank pneumonia can be rapid. Not giving these measures to an elderly patient is an oversight in post-operative care.

A normal enhanced recovery protocol will have set walking distances to be covered at given post-operative periods; this will prevent problems associated with prolonged bed rest, chest complications, bed sores, muscle wastage, bone resorption, constipation and thromboembolism. Whilst an elderly patient may not manage to walk an unaided 50 m 4 times on day 1 as would be 'prescribed' for a younger patient, an approach tailored to the individual should be followed, e.g. a previously mobile 85-year-old patient should walk an aided 15 m 4 times on day 1. Thus, the elderly can benefit from all facets of the enhanced recovery approach which should not be at a slower pace, rather tailored to the individual.

11.6   The Elderly Need Less Attention to Post-operative Pain

Good post-operative pain control whilst not only being a humane prerequisite has many advantages (allows mobility, prevents chest infection, prevents thromboembolism, limits the stress response, reduces ileus, etc.), hence is of importance for all. In actual fact, the elderly will require a lot more attention to optimize this than in a younger patient. The elderly will often be on a multitude of medication, these may interact with strong opioids, and opioids will also be poorly excreted/metabolized; hence, close attention, monitoring for signs of toxicity and dose adjustment may well be needed. The patient-controlled administration of analgesic (PCA) route is often used following major surgery; in the elderly, this may not be available either due to a lack of mental capacity or dexterity. In these settings, continuous infusions may be needed which will necessitate critical care observation. Epidural analgesia needs to be tailored appropriately due to access issues or hypotension. For these reasons, post-operative analgesia in the elderly patient can be an extremely complex area, and it is important to get it 'right'; hence, senior experienced anaesthetic input is of benefit.

11.7   All Specific Critical Care Targets Should Be Met

Traditionally, targets are set for certain haemodynamic parameters; clearly, it is sensible that these are tailored to an individual's usual preoperative blood pressure or pulse. Fluid balance is one area we have touched on in 11.5 and is often difficult to gauge in high-risk patients such as the elderly, balancing the risks of parenteral fluid versus dehydration and pre-renal failure. In the authors' opinion, it is far too frequently 'chased' aggressively to this group of patient's detriment. There is good evidence that cautious limitation of intravenous fluids leads to fewer complications and faster recovery (Lobo et al. 2002). The traditional 0.5 ml/kg lean body mass is often too higher target especially in this group of patients, chasing fluids not only risks cardiac failure but also causes third space losses with particular effects on the gut; this establishes a vicious circle where an ileus develops due to fluid overload; hence, patients vomit and therefore further high doses of intravenous fluid are given. So how can you assess if your elderly patient is getting adequate fluids? A lower target of 0.3 ml/kg is adequate alongside clinical assessment; having a warm periphery and normal cognitive function is a far more useful gauge of adequate perfusion. It is important anaesthetists and surgeons understand these concepts particularly for this group of patients as the risks of fluid overload and cardiac failure potentially with subsequent myocardial infarction are significant.

Many anaesthetists will have a blanket policy in using arterial and central lines in all elderly patients; however, insertion is not without complication and prolonged use will limit mobility and risk infection. Clearly, a balance has to be sought, and their use should be in a tailored fashion. If they are needed, then they should be removed, as with all lines, catheters and drains, as soon as possible.

Thus, specific critical care targets can act as guidelines but will need tailoring to the individual and do not always need to be met.

11.8   Elderly Patients' Nutritional Needs Will Often Be Met by Early Reintroduction of Diet

Whilst there is good evidence that early reintroduction of diet is of benefit as part of an enhanced recovery protocol (Varadhan et al. 2010a, b), this may not be sufficient for this group of patients. The elderly are more frequently at risk of malnutrition at presentation compared to younger patients; however, if adequate nutritional support is put in place, then an increase in post-operative complications does not necessarily follow (Jin et al. 2011). In the post-operative period, as for all, there is a risk of ileus and the enteral route may not be available; furthermore, in the elderly delirium, incapacity and poor coordination may also limit the reintroduction of diet. Careful assessment by dietitians should be in place along with good nursing care. All elderly patients should be assessed for malnutrition, and the use of scoring tools such as the MUST score (Stratton et al. 2004) is useful. Total parenteral nutrition should be available and used promptly where needed if there is evidence of gut failure and malnutrition.

11.9   Where Guidelines (e.g. NICE) and Protocols Exist They Should Be Adhered to Closely

There is a whole wealth of evidence-based guidance on post-operative care. It must be borne in mind, however, that it is usually based on normal adult populations with normal physiology. When we look at the elderly population, they are at increased risk of thromboembolism (CCCG 2000), and it is standard practice in the United Kingdom to use a multifaceted approach to reduce this risk (e.g. NICE guidance) (NICE 2010). Whilst it is imperative that risks of thromboembolism are reduced by measures such as smoking cessation and discontinuing hormone replacement, strict application of all prophylactic measures mentioned in any guidance may not be appropriate or indeed safe. For example, standard prophylaxis as mentioned in NICE guidance would include preoperative pneumatic calf compression, post-operative compression stockings (e.g. TED stockings) and pharmacological prophylaxis with low molecular weight heparin (LMWH). In an elderly population, there will frequently be impaired renal function such that dosing of LMWH may need to be reduced. Peripheral vascular disease will often co-exist. Safe practice would suggest that ankle brachial pressure indices be checked prior to application of mechanical calf compression with either pneumatic devices or stockings. Hence, whilst guidelines may exist, they should be used as just that, guidelines, and tailored to an individual patient.

11.10   Special Equipment Is Needed to Help Compensate for the Functional Disabilities of the Elderly

There is a well-recognized pathway progressing through functional decline, with a subsequent loss of independence resulting in institutionalized care (Quinn et al. 2011). It is imperative that all carers looking after elderly patients repeatedly assess and intervene with appropriate measures to aim to prevent this decline which is all too often *not* inevitable. Comprehensive geriatric assessment has a key role to play here and should be sought at the earliest opportunity. However, whilst patients may need certain 'aids' such as spectacles to see and read, it is important to fully assess what a patient does and indeed does not need. Forcing all manner of gadgets on a patient when they are not necessary only makes a patient withdraw and potentially decline further. Rehabilitation in the elderly should focus on shedding the need for compensatory gadgets rather than encourage their use. Often what elderly patients need in such scenarios is formal careful functional assessment with aggressive rehabilitation.

An example of this would be a previously mobile elderly patient who is struggling to walk after their operation. They have otherwise recovered well, and their wound pain is well controlled. A walking frame is given to the patient; however, the 'proud' patient sees this as an encumbrance and does not feel they will be able to cope at home with it. They do not voice this to their carers due to mild dementia which has been exacerbated by being away from their normal surroundings. It is not hard to see that this could easily lead to a severe functional decline such that the patient does not ever reach their previous levels of independence and ends up in institutional care. Often an adequate assessment with a multidisciplinary focus will reveal specific problems. In this case, it may be that the patient is not receiving their normal gout medication; hence, walking is difficult; they previously have needed aids to stand but once up are freely mobile. As a result of their operation, their lower limb, specifically calf strength, has diminished such that they cannot mobilize as before. The lack of hand aids to stand has been lacking. Good functional assessment and aggressive rehabilitation will identify and treat issues such as these and hopefully prevent this downward spiral (Quinn et al. 2011).

11.11 Post-operative Care Should Continue After Discharge

In many Western and Asian healthcare systems, there are often increasing financial burdens on hospitals. One area that has been looked at critically is outpatient follow-up after admission. Frequently, recommendations are made that patients should not have hospital follow-up; rather, it is left in the hands of the general practitioner. This approach can often leave elderly patients in a dangerous position. As discussed, elderly patients are at risk of functional decline in the immediate post-operative period, but it is important to recognize that these problems can still occur after discharge. Patients may well have to cope with many new challenges such as coping with stomas, drains, new medications and pain management. They may also not be able to be as 'independent' as before due to recuperation, tiredness and inability to drive for several weeks after major surgery. A framework of appropriate follow-up and home visits need to be in place to be receptive in this critical period such that all the previous efforts are not undone.

Conclusion

It is without doubt elderly patients are at more risk than a standard adult population; however, they are at more risk of general as opposed to surgical site-specific complications. Chest, cardiac and thromboembolic complications recurrently

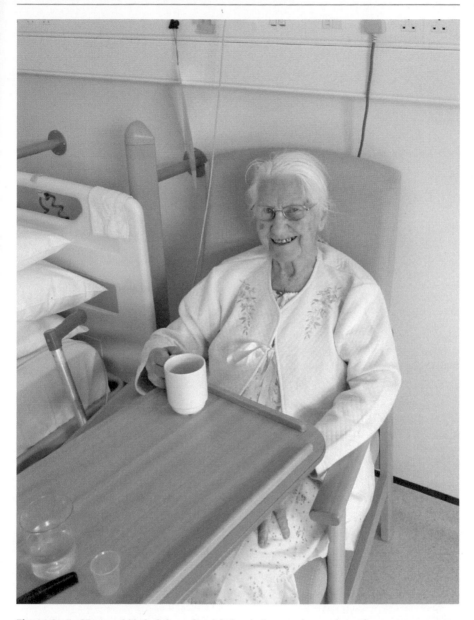

Fig. 11.2 An 87-year-old lady 2 days after right hemicolectomy in an enhanced recovery programme

present the biggest incidence of problems. Delirium is frequently seen, but if not preventable, its severity can often be lessened, and when it does occur, it is all too often poorly managed.

Elderly patients do require critical care input, but specifics need to be tailored to an elderly patient's usual physiology; this also applies to the application of standard adult guidelines. Whilst it is important to pay heed to specific surgical recovery, we have to remember what our ultimate aim is. This must be to return our elderly patients to a good quality of life and, where possible, an independent existence. Functional decline presents a huge risk to this, and a transdisciplinary approach should be followed to prevent this (Fig. 11.2).

References

Basili G, Lorenzetti L, Biondi G et al (2008) Colorectal cancer in the elderly. Is there a role for safe and curative surgery? ANZ J Surg 78:466–470

Cavaliere F, Conti G, Costa R et al (2008) Intensive care after elective surgery: a survey on 30-day postoperative mortality and morbidity. Minerva Anestesiol 74:459–468

Chee J, Tan KY (2010) Outcome studies on older patients undergoing surgery are missing the mark. J Am Geriatr Soc 58:2238–2239

Christmas C, Makary MA, Burton JR (2006) Medical considerations in older surgical patients. J Am Coll Surg 203:746–751

Colorectal cancer collaborative group (2000) Surgery for colorectal cancer in elderly patients: a systematic review. Lancet 356:968–974

Doyle RL (1999) Assessing and modifying the risk of postoperative pulmonary complications. Chest 115:77–81

Gouvas N, Tan E, Windsor A et al (2009) Fast-track vs standard care in colorectal surgery: a meta-analysis update. Int J Colorectal Dis 24:1119–1131

Halter J, Ouslander J, Tinetti M (2009) Hazzard's geriatric medicine and gerontology. McGraw-Hill, New York

Jin L, Inoue N, Sato N et al (2011) Comparison between surgical outcomes of colorectal cancer in younger and elderly patients. World J Gastroenterol 28:1642–1648

Lobo DN, Bostock KA, Neal KR et al (2002) Effect of salt and water balance on recovery of gastrointestinal function after elective colonic resection: a randomised controlled trial. Lancet 25:1812–1818

Marusch F, Koch A, Schmidt U et al (2005) The impact of the risk factor "age" on the early postoperative results of surgery for colorectal carcinoma and its significance for perioperative management. World J Surg 29:1013–1022

NICE (2010) Venous thromboembolism: reducing the risk. National institute for health and clinical excellence. http://guidance.nice.org.uk/CG92

Pedrazzani C, Cerullo G, De Marco G et al (2009) Impact of age-related comorbidity of colorectal cancer surgery. World J Gastroenterol 15(45):5706–5711

Quinn TJ, Mcarthur K, Ellis G et al (2011) Functional assessment in older people. BMJ 343(7821):469–473

Stratton RJ, Hackston A, Longmore D et al (2004) Malnutrition in hospital outpatients and inpatients: prevalence, concurrent validity and ease of use of the 'malnutrition universal screening tool' ('MUST') for adults. Br J Nutr 92:799–808

Tan E, Tilney H, Thompson M (2007) The United Kingdom National Bowel Cancer Project-epidemiology and surgical risk in the elderly. Eur J Cancer 43:2285–2294

Tan KY, Chen CN, Ng C et al (2006) Which octogenarians do poorly after major open abdominal surgery in our Asian population? World J Surg 30:547–552

Tan KY, Kawamura Y, Mizokami K et al (2009) Colorectal surgery in octogenarian patients – outcomes and predictions of morbidity. Int J Colorectal Dis 24:185–189

Tan KY, Konishi F, Tan L et al (2010) Optimizing the management of elderly colorectal surgery patients. Surg Today 40:999–1010

Varadhan KK, Lobo DN et al (2010a) Enhanced recovery after surgery: the future of improving surgical care. Crit Care Clin 26:527–547

Varadhan KK, Neal KR, Dejong CH et al (2010b) The enhanced recovery after surgery (ERAS) pathway for patients undergoing major elective open colorectal surgery: a meta-analysis of randomized controlled trials. Clin Nutr 29:434–440

Nursing Care of the Elderly Surgical Patients

12

Phyllis Xiu-Zhuang Tan and Gek-Choo Chua

Take Home Pearls

- Nurses play a vital role in providing multifaceted care through an effective trans-disciplinary team.
- Patient and family education is of utmost importance in preparing the minds psychologically and alleviating the fears that predisposes an elderly to post-operative delirium.
- Consistent, patient and empathic nursing care through excellent communication, patient engagement and uncompromising attention to detail are the cornerstones of excellent nursing care of an elderly surgical patient.

12.1 Introduction

The importance of specialized nursing in an elderly surgical patient is driven by the fact that age advancement predisposes an elderly surgical patient to higher risk of surgery. This is because of age-related physiological changes which include decrease in cognition, cardiac, respiratory, renal functions and other co-morbid conditions. The declining physiological reserves that may be used to maintain the normal homeostasis of the ageing body may not be sufficient to meet the increased demands in the event of an acute illness and surgical stress (Tan et al. 2010). The physical phenotype may be manifested in patients defined as frail in current concepts.

P.X.-Z. Tan (✉) • G.-C. Chua
Department of Nursing Administration, Alexandra Health Private Limited,
Khoo Teck Puat Hospital, Singapore, Singapore
e-mail: tan.phyllis.xz@alexandrahealth.com.sg;chua.gek.choo@alexandrahealth.com.sg

K.-Y. Tan (ed.), *Colorectal Cancer in the Elderly*,
DOI 10.1007/978-3-642-29883-7_12, © Springer-Verlag Berlin Heidelberg 2013

Fig. 12.1 Concept of
multifaceted care

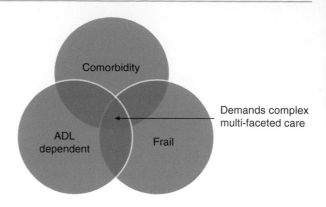

An elderly patient may also have decline in the visual, touch and hearing senses. This increases the challenge of nursing care. Co-morbidities, dependence on activities of daily living and frailty are interrelated and overlapping (Fig. 12.1). These interplaying factors work to demand multifaceted care in an elderly surgical patient. Physical, functional and emotional recovery of the geriatric patient undergoing major colorectal surgery cannot depend on merely the mastery skills of the surgeon alone. Multifaceted care has to be delivered through an effective interdisciplinary team in which the nurse plays a vital role. Nurses need to equip themselves with the additional skills and knowledge to provide the quality care required to facilitate such a care model in this complex group of geriatric patients. It involves planning and engaging in the care that addresses the special needs of the elderly patient (Ergina et al. 1993). In this chapter, the considerations for nursing care of the elderly surgical patients will be discussed.

12.2   Pre-operative Nursing Considerations

The components of pre-operative nursing include the need to establish the lines of communication which is essential before all other important components can be achieved. The provision of adequate psychological support, patient and family education and engagement are crucial for patients to be equipped with the knowledge and autonomy to engage themselves in the recovery process.

12.2.1 Establishing Communication Lines

Effective communication and rapport must be established before education can take place. Good patient-nurse communication and relationship facilitate better understanding and compliance towards the surgery and post-operative care.

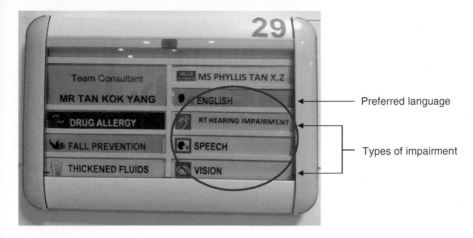

Fig. 12.2 Patient's information panel

The level of communication is tailored to the cognitive and intellectual status of each unique individual. Limitations from age-related physiological changes are taken into consideration. Sensory losses, decline in thought processes and memory lapses hinder effective communication. Patients with slower cognitive function demand extra time and patience. Individuals with visual impairment may need their visual aids and education materials to be printed in larger fonts to allow them to see and understand, while those with hearing deficit may require hearing aids or other modes of communication such as writing instead of speaking. Words and sentences must be simplified and conveyed in a clear, slow and low tone of voice, in a language preferred by the geriatric patient. This will promote effective listening.

When nursing staff are handing over the care to another team, it is essential to convey the best mode of communication between the new nursing team and the anxious elderly patient. Failure in communications may result in accidental injuries from the patient's attempt to achieve their unmet needs. The use of a patient information panel (Fig. 12.2) at the bedside is one measure that can be used to convey the special needs of an individual including their means of communication at one glance. This may facilitate more effective communication for healthcare team members especially those who are seeing the elderly patient for the first time.

It is important to note that effective communication needs to be established prior to surgery so that it can be maintained in the post-operative period. This will then facilitate effective communication and provision of nursing care when the patient feels more discomfort after major surgery.

12.2.2 Psychological Preparedness

The trauma of major surgery is a significant stressor for most elderly patients and their families. Common sources of fear in a geriatric surgery patient include the following:
1. Pain
2. Loss of independence and/or not being in control
3. Burden to family members
4. Death following a major surgery at an advanced age
5. Separation from family and loved ones
6. Fear of the unknown

The psychological condition of a geriatric patient undergoing major surgery can have a stronger influence than the physical condition. Suboptimal psychological preparation can increase the risk of delirium which can potentially result in an overall negative impact during their hospitalization. Therefore, it is important for the healthcare team to address this fear effectively which can be done through frequent reassurance from the team and through patient education where expected peri-operative experiences are advised.

12.2.2.1 Patient and Family Education

Patient and family education is an ongoing process that is reinforced throughout the peri-operative period and serves to manage the patients' expectations on the recovery process (Tan et al. 2010). It is of utmost importance in preparing the minds psychologically and alleviating the fears of both the elderly surgical patients and their loved ones. It shall be done pre-operatively in the absence of other compounding stressors and distractions such as pain, effects of medications and other factors that may accompany most major surgeries.

The nurse provides the educational package following the surgeon's consultation. Establishing the readiness of patients to learn is essential before education takes place. Information pertaining to the surgery and expected responsibilities from the patients are advised so that they can anticipate and actively involve themselves in the recovery process. The patients and families are encouraged to express themselves and clarify doubts during the education session so that the healthcare team can assist to address the concerns of each individual.

Age-related changes can affect the elderly patient's ability to learn new material; therefore, modification of traditional teaching approaches shall be used to enhance effectiveness (Tan et al. 2010). Creative educational adjuncts can be used to promote interest and enhance learning for both patients and their family members. Some examples include:
1. *Presentation slides consisting of information relevant to the recovery process*
These slides are used by the nurse clinician as she provides verbal explanation in the language preferred by the unique individual.
2. *Information sheets (Appendix A.1)*
A simplified summary of the daily progress and information sheets are issued to patients as a guide. This allows them to anticipate the type of care that will be prescribed

by the healthcare team in accordance to their recovery progress and the activities that they should be engaged in.

3. *Video testimonies*

Patients with similar conditions who have had operations done are shown to reassure them of the high possibility of a good surgical outcome. This is to provide them with a more positive outlook on their surgery and to motivate them in early engagement of rehabilitative activities post-operatively.

4. *Adjuncts*

The use of educational adjuncts will allow better visual understanding. The patients who require a stoma will be provided with a set of ostomy appliance after the pre-operative education. This will allow them the opportunity for hands-on practice at home and reduce the stress from learning post-operatively. Areas that need improvement will be reinforced by the nurse clinician prior to discharge.

12.2.2.2 Patient Engagement

Patients need to be engaged to take action for their own well-being. Elderly patients often lose their ability to be in control of their own health decisions whenever they are admitted to the healthcare institution. Nurses play an important role in encouraging elderly surgical patients to be more empowered in their own recovery process during the peri-operative period (Tan et al. 2010).

In the Asian context, family members tend to take over the responsibility in liaising and decision making of treatment plans with the healthcare team, leaving the elderly with the only treatment option that is decided by their loved ones. Patients also feel that they have to leave every aspect of care to the healthcare professional, when actually their motivation and input have a profound effect. Patients who are engaged in taking actions for their own well-being are more likely to adhere to chosen courses of treatment and participate in activities to aid recovery (Coulter 2007). Thus, in the context of geriatric surgery, involving the patients and respecting their decision for or against various aspects of the treatment process (e.g. prolonged intubation) should take top priority.

Realistic goals are set with the patients to manage their expectations effectively and improve their motivation to participate in rehabilitative activities. Some examples of patient engagement during the peri-operative period include nutritional optimization where the informed patients diligently adhere to the diet plan understanding the implications of non-compliance. They also actively participate in individualized physical and respiratory exercises prescribed by the physiotherapist. All these lower the risk of developing complications associated with prolonged confinement to bed such as atelectasis, deep vein thrombosis and functional decline that can inhibit their recovery process. Patients who require a stoma start practicing stoma care with the appliances that are provided before the surgery. This facilitates early participation in self care and improves confidence for discharge.

An example is an 84-year-old Qigong (Chinese Martial Arts) Master (Madam Lee) with 36 disciples. She was diagnosed to have localized cancer of the colon and needed surgery. The management plan was discussed extensively with her and her family. Her main hesitation towards surgery was the fear of not being able to return to her daily Qigong and continue to teach her disciples. Being very independent she did not want to be in a state where she would be dependent on her family. The goal of returning to Qigong after surgery was set with Madam Lee. Pre-operative education was provided with presentation slides and video testimonies. She realized how important it was to be engaged in rehabilitative activities during the peri-operative period so as to achieve her goal. Thus, she participated actively in the rehabilitative activities that were started from the first post-operative day, facilitated by the nursing staff and surgical care team. She was subsequently able to demonstrate a sequence of Qigong to the healthcare team 1 week after colectomy. She subsequently returned to her daily Qigong routine and teaching after 6 weeks of rehabilitation.

Discharge planning before the surgery can prevent unnecessary prolonged stay that can predispose the elderly patients to nosocomial infections. It involves the identification of the main caregivers as well as discussion of the potential need for short-term stay at step-down hospitals for rehabilitation. Pre-emptive referrals can be made to shorten the waiting time for bed availability. This will allow ample time for the family members to anticipate and make arrangements among themselves before the patient is discharged to an environment that is safe for recuperation. Constant update of patient's condition and management plans to family members provides directions that are in accordance with the healthcare team. Patients are also frequently asked about their feelings throughout their hospitalization so that the team can assist in addressing any of their concerns promptly.

Table 12.1 summarizes the ways of engaging patients and families during the peri-operative period.

12.2.3 Nutritional Consideration

Malnutrition is a common problem in the ageing population, and it is often caused by various factors such as socio-economic status, health factor, poor dentition, poor physical functional level and knowledge deficit (Potter and Perry 1997). In the geriatric patient who is undergoing major surgery, nutrition helps to maintain the physical well-being that is essential for recovery and wound healing during the peri-operative period.

Table 12.1 Ways to promote patient and family engagement in geriatric surgery	1. Discuss treatment plans and decision making with the patients and their family
	2. Set clear goals for treatment
	3. Plan for discharge before surgery to prevent unnecessary prolonged hospitalization
	4. Encourage the geriatric surgical patient to participate in rehabilitative activities
	5. Encourage family participation in providing comfort and emotional support
	6. Empathize through listening
	7. Provide an open door communication between the healthcare team, patient and family

One would think optimizing the nutritional level of the elderly surgical patient is solely the role of the dietitian. However, nurses play an extremely important role in identifying the patients who are at risk of malnutrition and ensuring they receive the optimized nutritional plan prescribed by the dietitian.

The holistic assessment of all geriatric surgical patients by the nurse serves as a guide to identify and provide interventions to address factors that can compromise the treatment plan. For instance, screening for the risk of malnutrition using the nutritional assessment tool (Appendix A.2) allows the nurse and dietitian to identify high-risk patients. The transdisciplinary team can then determine the need for longer periods of nutritional optimization prior to elective surgery. The nurse who identifies the patient with poor socio-economic support can also communicate with the medical social worker to address financial concerns.

There is also a need for the nurse to ensure that the oral condition of patients does not adversely affect their ability to consume the recommended diet. The availability of well-fitted dentures and good oral hygiene are some factors that can affect the oral intake of geriatric patients.

12.3   Post-Operative Considerations

Effective nursing care to complement good surgery involves the observational and critical thinking skills of the nurse. It includes vigilant monitoring of these geriatric surgical patients and the ability to react promptly to any subtle changes during the initial post-operative period.

Changes in the vital signs and behaviour may suggest signs of complications. Nurses should take pride in the accuracy of fluid input and output charts as this is vital for precise tailoring of fluid management that is so vital in the elderly.

Besides the monitoring of vital signs, input and output of the elderly patients, nursing care includes the provision of a safe and therapeutic environment.

12.3.1 Pain Management

The concern of using potent analgesics and the misconception that pain sensations are diminished in older people often result in inadequate pain control (Tan et al. 2010). Several studies suggest that the incidence of delirium is reduced when pain is appropriately managed (Potter and Perry 1997). Pain, if not well optimized, can affect the patient's participation in post-operative rehabilitative activities as well.

The nurse ensures analgesics are administered timely and pain assessment is carried out regularly with appropriate tools tailored for each different individual. The pain assessment tools that are commonly used include the following:

The numeric pain scale (Fig. 12.3) is used for patients who are more intellectual and are well versed with the usage instructions from the nurse. Patients will be asked to grade their severity of pain from a score of zero indicating no pain to a score of ten representing the worst imaginable pain.

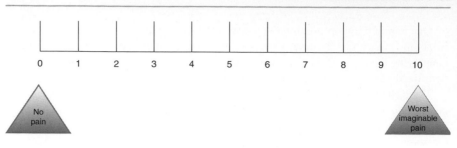

Fig. 12.3 Numeric pain scale

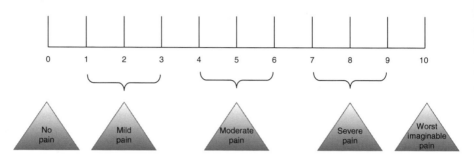

Fig. 12.4 Descriptive pain scale

The descriptive scale is more commonly used in the geriatric population who are not able to provide a precise pain score. They will be asked to describe their pain severity in terms of no pain, mild pain, moderate pain, severe pain and worst imaginable pain. The range of score for each category of pain is reflected in Fig. 12.4.

The facial pain scale (Fig. 12.5) is used in patients with some sensory deficit such as hearing or speech impairment. They will be asked to point out the facial expression that best describes their pain.

Interventions need to be implemented according to the pain severity reported by the patient.

Table 12.2 serves as a guide for nursing staff to initiate intervention in accordance to the pain score for the three commonly used pain assessment tools. The re-evaluation of pain using the same tool following an intervention is important to assess for the efficacy of medications. Variations in the use of pain assessment tools should be avoided for accuracy and consistency. Pain scores are clearly documented for careful and effective prescription of analgesics.

Besides the use of pharmacological interventions to relief pain, nurses can use non-pharmacological interventions such as providing a comfortable position and a comfort pillow to support the surgical site following a major abdominal surgery. Distraction methods such as playing of soothing music and book reading are other methods of non-pharmacological interventions in pain management.

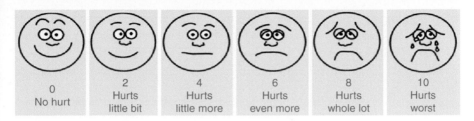

Fig. 12.5   Facial pain scale (Adapted from Wong 1988)

Table 12.2   Pain relieve intervention guide

Pain intensity score by patient				
Numeric	Descriptive		Faces	Intervention
0	No pain	0	0	None
1–3	Mild pain	2	2	Serve analgesics around the clock as prescribed
4–6	Moderate pain	5	5	Discuss pain management plan with team if necessary
7–9	Severe pain	8	8	Inform doctor to see urgently and review treatment
10	Worst pain	10	10	Inform doctor to see urgently and review treatment

Adapted from Khoo Teck Puat Hospital, Alexandra Health, Singapore

12.3.2 Hypoxia

Respiratory compromise may occur in an elderly patient following general anaesthesia together with use of intravenous or regional opioids during the initial postoperative period. The geriatric surgical patient should be nursed with supplemental oxygen therapy and monitored for signs of desaturation in oxygenation levels. The head of bed should be propped up to at least 30° to promote chest wall expansion for more effective gas exchange. Oral suction may be performed in patients who are unable to expectorate on their own.

12.3.3 Tubes and Lines

The presence of tubes such as indwelling catheter, abdominal drains and central venous catheters is common after a major colorectal surgery. Nursing care of these patients will include ensuring all tubes and lines are serving their appropriate purpose. Drainage tube observation should not just be of output volume but also include the nature of drainage fluid. For example, if a sudden increase in the amount of fresh red blood from the abdominal drains is evident, that may suggest an intra-abdominal bleed needing emergent attention. The nursing team also should ensure tubes and lines are well secured to prevent accidental dislodgement especially in elderly patients who are at risk of developing delirium or cognitive dysfunction. Nurses should play an active role in reviewing the tubes with the team doctors. Tubes and lines should be removed as early as possible to minimize the risk of infection. The absence of tubes and lines also promote better comfort and facilitate mobilization.

12.3.4 Early Mobilization

Complications such as atelectasis, deep vein thrombosis, deconditioning of muscles and joint functions, development of pressure ulcers, constipation and incontinence are often associated with prolonged confinement to bed. The rehabilitative aspects of care are often left to the physiotherapists. The nurse should play an active role in encouraging the patients to participate in exercises prescribed by physiotherapists. The patients should be encouraged to sit out of bed several times throughout the day and perform deep breathing exercises for effective gas exchange of the lungs. This can aid in the prevention of chest infection.

The nursing staff should encourage supervised ambulation at ward level as much as possible. Some ways to do so include encouraging the patient to ambulate to the washroom for shower where they can engage themselves in their activities of daily living at the same time, or voiding purposes instead of agreeing to the common requests for bed bath and urinal or bedpan. Family members can be involved in the rehabilitative activities such as helping the patients with passive limb exercises to promote blood circulation and prevention of muscle wastage when patient is resting in bed. When deemed safe, family members should be encouraged to ambulate with the geriatric surgical patients during their visitation.

Nurses should proactively provide the physiotherapists with accurate feedback of patients' rehabilitative progress and the team's management plan so that they can tailor the plan for rehabilitation in accordance to the tolerance level of each individual. The ability to start mobilizing in the early post-operative period provides patients with the assurance of regaining their independence and functional status. This will increase the motivation in engaging themselves in rehabilitation that aids early functional recovery.

12.3.5 Unfamiliar Environment

Frequent ward and/or bed transfers should be avoided as an unfamiliar environment often results in disorientation and increases the risk of acute confusion in an elderly patient. Bed allocation for elderly surgical patients should be within the vicinity of the nursing counter to allow for better observation and easy access in getting the attention from the nursing staff. Frequent visitation of family members should be encouraged and not be restricted to visiting hours only. They should be encouraged to bring items that the geriatric patients are familiar with as a "security blanket" to provide them with the comfort and sense of security. Some of these examples are photographs of loved ones, hairbands and pillows that the patient sleeps with. The room that patients are nursed in should be well ventilated with adequate windows and a clock with large number prints to provide them with the orientation to different times of the day. The attempt to create an environment similar to that of their home minimizes the risk of delirium and cognitive dysfunction.

12.3.6 Hearing or Visual Impairment

The senses of hearing and vision play important roles in the orientation of the geriatric surgical patients. Nursing staff should always ensure that patients with hearing and visual impairment have their aids at all times. The awareness of surrounding environmental situations can prevent injuries related to fall that may result from suboptimal vision. Hearing the progress, treatment plans and assurance that allays the anxiety during the post-operative period can reduce the risk of post-operative delirium and cognitive dysfunction.

12.3.7 Sleep Deprivation

Lack of adequate rest can contribute to delirium or cognitive dysfunction. During the initial period, the geriatric patient may experience sleep disturbance due to various factors such as frequent monitoring of vital signs and pain. Nursing care should be coordinated so that the patients' rest will be least interrupted. For instance, serving of medications can be scheduled at timings that coincide with the intervals of vital signs monitoring or just before bedtime. Gentle reminders can be made to the team to review the frequency of vital signs monitoring for patients with a stable trend recorded overnight.

The patients who have had their urinary catheter removed should be encouraged to empty their bladder and discouraged from drinking water just before they sleep to minimize the frequency to void at night. Effort should be made to dim down lights and minimize noise levels to provide a conducive resting environment when activities are minimal at night. These measures will promote better sleep pattern and prevent sleep deprivation.

12.3.8 Eliminating Disturbance

It is common for the elderly to experience bowel disturbance with a shortened intestinal tract following a colon resection. The patient may find an increase in the need for passage of watery stools during the initial period. The nurse should monitor bowel movements and encourage adequate fluid intake if not contraindicated to maintain fluid balance. The increase in fluid intake may also result in an increase in the need for urination. The geriatric surgical patient should be nursed in a room with adequate lighting in the day and easy access to toilet facilities to prevent potential accidents such as falls that can occur from frequent visits to the bathroom. There is a need for the nurse to be vigilant for signs of delirium. Frequent passage of watery stools can result in electrolyte imbalances contributing to delirium if not corrected.

12.4 Post-operative Delirium

Geriatric patients undergoing major surgery are at risk of post-operative delirium and cognitive dysfunction. These may lead to falls, wound problems, dislodged tubes and aspiration (Tan et al. 2010).

Patients are often restrained for their safety to prevent them from sustaining injuries during an episode of delirium. This may aggravate frustration and may result in more aggressive behaviours in patients' attempt to "escape from the false imprisonment". Unnecessary restraining should not be incorporated as part of the nursing intervention. A checklist (Appendix A.3) of risk factors for delirium in the geriatric surgical patients can be used. Interventions can then be implemented.

Conclusion

Nurses play vital roles in the transdisciplinary care of complex geriatric surgery patients. Being the healthcare professional who have the most frequent contact with patients, nurses shall provide consistent, patient and compassionate care through excellent communication, patient engagement and uncompromising attention to detail. These are the cornerstones of excellent nursing care of an elderly surgical patient. An engaged patient would enhance compliance to treatment, thus enhancing rehabilitation and recovery from the major surgery. Nurses should relish this challenge in an era of extraordinary empowerment.

Appendices

Appendix A.1: Guide for Patients Undergoing Colorectal Surgery

	Operation day	POD 1	POD 2 POD 3 - 4	POD 5 – 7
Medications	Fluids will be given through your veins for hydration. Medications will be given to you for: – Pain relief – Preventing nausea/vomiting after operation – For preventing infection if needed	Oral painkillers will be ordered. Fluids will continue to be given through your veins until you can drink orally.	Pain assessment will be done by our doctors and medications will be prescribed accordingly. Fluids given through the veins will be adjusted according to: – Output from the tubes – Blood pressure, heart rate – Urine output – Blood results – Oral intake	Apart from your usual medications (if any), oral painkillers will be prescribed for you to take when necessary.

	Operation day POD 1	POD 2	POD 3 - 4	POD 5 – 7
Treatment / Management	Oxygen will be given through a tubing placed at your nostrils (nose). Presence of multiple tubes: – Small flexible tube inserted into your vein for fluids and medication to be given – Abdominal drain – Urine tube – Tube inserted through the anus. Blood tests may be ordered after operation. Wound dressings will only be changed upon doctor's order. Socks to prevent clotting of blood in the legs will be obtained.	Oxygen will be weaned off gradually. Urine tube may be removed. Please report to nursing staff whenever you need to void after removal of urine tube.	Tubes may be removed on doctor's order. Your doctor will inform you of the care plan and day of discharge.	You will be assessed for fitness for discharge. Wound dressings will be removed and left exposed if dry. Wound care advice will be reinforced. Stitches/ clips may be removed on the 10th day after operation at the polyclinic.

Monitoring

	Operation day	POD 1	POD 2	POD 3 – 4	POD 5 – 7
	You may be transferred to a special care area for close observation after operation. Hourly monitoring will be carried on the following: – Blood pressure – Pulse rate – Respiratory rate – Urine output	You will be reviewed by surgeons twice a day or as indicated for: – Lungs assessment – Temperature, blood pressure, heart rate, breathing rate and pain level. – Amount of fluids from tubes (if any) – Wound dressing – Readiness for progression of food intake. – Passage of flatus/ gas and stools/ motion after operation.			

Nutrition

	Operation day	POD 1	POD 2	POD 3 – 4	POD 5 – 7
	No food and drinks orally but may allow sips of water before surgery. You may be allowed some oral fluids after operation.	Clear feeds will usually be allowed. Some may be allowed liquid diet.	You may be put on liquid diet to low fiber soft diet. Please inform the doctor/ nurse if you feel any bloatedness/ discomfort in your abdomen after taking liquid diet.	Liquid diet to low fiber soft diet	Initial introduction of solid food will be low in fiber. Your surgeon/ nurse will advice you when ready for consumption of any food of your choice.

	Operation day	POD 1	POD 2	POD 3 - 4 POD 5 – 7
Activities	Passive limb exercises when in bed post-operatively to promote blood circulation. Breathing exercises when awake to promote lung expansion and prevent chest complications.	Physiotherapist will assist you in rehabilitative activities as follow: – Sitting out of bed – Deep breathing exercises – Effecting coughing technique – Passive limb exercises	You are expected to start ambulation with assistance by today. – Physiotherapist /nurses will assist you in returning to pre-operative baseline functional status.	Daily physiotherapist review till independent mobility is achieved.

	Operation day	POD 1	POD 2	POD 3 - 4	POD 5 – 7
Hygiene	You may take a shower before operation.	Nursing staff will assist you in maintaining hygiene at bedside.		You will be assisted by nursing staff to bathroom for shower.	You may ambulate on your own if deem fit for personal hygiene and cleanliness.

	Operation day	POD 1	POD 2	POD 3 - 4	POD 5 – 7
Communication	Your surgeons will update operative findings to you and family members.	On-going updates of conditions and treatment plans will be communicated to u and family. Nursing staff will educate you on post-operative care.			

Please note that the above are only guidelines and should be varied in accordance to meet individual patient's needs.

Appendix A.2: Nutritional Assessment Tool

Criteria / Score	Diseases with risks of malnutrition (Tick 1 or more)	Oral intake (Past 1 week) (Tick 1 only)	Unintentional weight loss (Past 6 months)	BMI (kg/m2) (Tick 1 only)
3	☐ Cancer ☐ AIDS ☐ Severe Burns ☐ Major Trauma ☐ Psychological ☐ Pressure Sores/ Wound ☐ End Stage Diseases ☐ Gastrointestinal Diseases (mal-absorption, ileus, obstruction, fistula) ☐ Sepsis / Severe Infection	☐ NBM or <1/4 share per meal ☐ Tube feeding < 1L/day (1 kcal/ml feed)	☐ >5kg	☐ <17.0
2	☐ Gastrointestinal Diseases (Others) ☐ Nutritional Anaemia	☐ 1/4 to < 3/4 share per meal ☐ Tube feeding < 1.5L/day (1 kcal/ml feed)	☐ < 5kg ☐ Yes, Unsure	☐ 17.0 to 18.5
1	☐ Uncomplicated Medical Condition With No Interruption in Food Intake	☐ 3/4 to 1 share per meal ☐ Tube feeding > 1.5L/day (1 kcal/ml feed)	☐ < 1kg ☐ No Change	☐ >18.5
Scoring	3 2 1	3 2 1	3 2 1	3 2 1
Total Score	(Refer to dietitian if score is 7 or more)			

PART 1: MODIFIED BURKE DYSPHAGIA SCREENING TOOL (Please tick the appropriate boxes)			
	Assessment of Risk Factors	Absent	Present
1	History of Stroke		
2	History of Pneumonia associated with acute stroke phase		
3	Cough associated with feeding		
4	Prolonged time required for feeding / swallowing		

NOTE:
- If 1 or more risk factors, refer Speech Therapist. Referral not required if patient is on long term tube feeding.
- No Risk Factors, complete Part 2.

No	PART 2: EXCLUSION CRITERIA FOR SWALLOWING ASSESSMENT	Please tick appropriate boxes
1	No difficulty in swallowing	
2	Able to take 2 or more meals without difficulties	
3	Patient on Stroke pathway	
4	Patient on NBM / PEG / NG tube	
	If yes to one or more criteria, OMIT Swallowing Assessment	

(Adapted from Khoo Teck Puat Hospital, Alexandra Health, Singapore)

Appendix A.3: Delirium Preventive Checklist

Delirium Preventive Measures
1. **Assessment of risk factors for post-operative delirium**
   - ☐ Pre-existing dementia
   - ☐ Poor nutritional status
   - ☐ Dehydration
   - ☐ Hearing or visual impairment
   - ☐ Hypoxia
   - ☐ Electrolyte imbalance (post-operatively)
   - ☐ Pain
   - ☐ Sleep deprivation
   - ☐ Elimination disturbances (bowel/urinary)
   - ☐ Presence of lines
   - ☐ Polypharmacy
   - ☐ Unfamiliar environment
   - ☐ Immobilization
2. **Preventive measures**
   - ☐ **Early mobilisation (from POD 1)**
     - ○ Physiotherapist involvement
     - ○ Review fall precaution (POD 3) and encourage ambulation
   - ☐ **Non-pharmacological measures**
     - ○ Pre-operative orientation
     - ○ Family involvement
     - ○ Environmental:
       - ☐ Review need for urine catheter (POD 2)
       - ☐ Pain control (POD 1)
       - ☐ Encourage voiding before bedtime (when catheter is removed)
       - ☐ Avoid restrainers
   - ☐ **Early intervention for dehydration and correct electrolyte imbalance**
   - ☐ **Oxygen therapy post-operatively**
   - ☐ **Avoid sleep deprivation**
     - ○ Reduce noise level at night
     - ○ Dim lights at bedtime
     - ○ Coordinate care to avoid interrupting sleep
     - ○ Review parameters schedule

Establish communication methods and adaptive equipment before surgery
Specify special needs (if any): _____

References

Coulter A (2007) When should you involve patients in treatment decisions? Br J Gen Pract 57(543):771–772
Ergina PL, Gold SL, Meakins JL (1993) Perioperative care of the elderly patient. World J Surg 17(2):192–198
Potter PA, Perry AG (1997) Fundamentals of nursing, 5th edn. Mosby, St. Louis
Tan KY, Konishi F, Tan L, Chin WK, Ong HY, Tan P (2010) Optimizing the management of elderly colorectal surgery patients. Surg Today 40(11):999–1010
Wong D (1988) Wong-Baker faces pain rating scale. [online-series]. Available at: http://www.wongbakerfaces.org. Accessed 27 Jan 2012

Returning to Premorbid Function After Colorectal Surgery in the Elderly

13

Kylie Ka-Fai Siu, Barbara Chun-Sian Wee,
Candice Kai-Ni Yeo, Clare Mullarkey,
Gregory Jia-Chyi Fam, and Sharon Cheng-Kuan Lim

Take Home Pearls

- The ageing process entails physical and physiological changes that place the person at higher risk of functional decline post-surgery.
- Common physical impairments include secretion retention, reduced lung volumes and acute physical deconditioning.
- The above are highly reversible states and can be addressed through physiotherapeutic interventions.
- Chest physiotherapy and early mobilisation remains the mainstay of management of the post-operative patient. These are even more critical in elderly persons where deterioration is more pronounced with longer bed rest and immobility.

13.1 Background

Post-operative complications are not uncommon. These complications include pain, reduced lung volumes, secretion retention, post-operative pneumonia, deep vein thrombosis and acute physical deconditioning. The development of these complications is largely due to the effects of general anaesthesia, post-operative associated pain and prolonged bed rest. Challenged by the physiological changes of ageing, elderly patients undergoing surgery, including colorectal surgery, are at higher risk

---

K.K.-F. Siu • B.C.-S. Wee • C.K.-N. Yeo • C. Mullarkey
G.J.-C. Fam • S.C.-K. Lim (✉)
Department of Rehabilitation Services, Khoo Teck Puat Hospital,
Alexandra Health, Singapore, Singapore
e-mail: lim.sharon.ck@alexandrahealth.com.sg

K.-Y. Tan (ed.), *Colorectal Cancer in the Elderly*,
DOI 10.1007/978-3-642-29883-7_13, © Springer-Verlag Berlin Heidelberg 2013

of these complications. From a physiotherapist's perspective, the above complications, while common and not unexpected, are highly preventable and reversible.

This chapter will discuss physiotherapy in the management of the elderly patient undergoing colorectal surgery in three parts:

1. The problem with surgery from a physiotherapy perspective
2. The problem with ageing and associated risks of post-operative complications
3. Physiotherapeutic interventions in the management of elderly patients who have undergone surgery

13.2   The Problem with Colorectal Surgery

The most important inspiratory muscle is the diaphragm. Research has shown that diaphragmatic excursion after abdominal surgery is reduced (Denehy 2008). Furthermore, post-operative pain may also contribute to diaphragmatic dysfunction. After abdominal surgery, these patients may also have the fear of stressing the surgical site such that breathing becomes shallow and/or apical. The use of general anaesthesia also causes changes in lung mechanics which may lead to a reduced functional residual capacity (FRC). This reduction, which may persist for 5–10 days, may be as great as 70% of the preoperative value, with the greatest reduction in the first and second post-operative day (Denehy 2008; Craig 1981). The closing capacity (CC) of an individual's lung volume also needs to be taken into consideration. When FRC is reduced and CC is increased, dependent airways begin to close or stop ventilating, resulting in dependent atelectasis, increased work of breathing and reduction in oxygenation (Denehy 2008).

13.3   The Problems of Ageing

Sarcopenia, the phenomenon of degenerative loss of skeletal muscle in the elderly, leads to overall reduction in strength and endurance. This has been correlated to mobility disorders, disability (Cruz-Jentoft et al. 2010) and henceforth functional decline.

In addition, the elderly tend to have higher prevalence of co-morbidities including cardiopulmonary and neurological diseases. These multiple co-morbidities can potentially limit functional reserve and exercise capacity, thereby contributing to higher incidences of functional decline (Cruz-Jentoft et al. 2010).

It has been shown that during hospitalisation and after discharge, older patients are at greater risk of developing functional decline (Van Craen et al. 2010). Functional decline can be further contributed to by previous falls, functional impairment, cognitive impairment or dementia, prior hospitalisation, incident vascular event, depression, vision impairment, diabetes mellitus and impaired mobility (Inouye et al. 2007). Through early identification of these risk factors, occurrences of functional decline can be reduced. From the physiotherapy point of view, interventions can be targeted at these impairments to delay further decline of function.

Ageing is associated with stiffening of vertebral and costovertebral joints, changes in spinal curvatures like increase in thoracic kyphosis and/or scoliosis, and changes in muscle and other soft tissue lengths. These can reduce chest wall compliance. This limits effective diaphragmatic contraction leading to incomplete lung emptying and increase air trapping. Due to the overall reduction in mechanical efficiency of the respiratory system, there is a significant increase in oxygen demand at any given level of exercise, and hence reduced exercise capacity (Berend 2005). Mucociliary clearance and cough reflex sensitivity has been shown to be more impaired amongst the elderly (Berend 2005). This impacts effective sputum expectoration for maintaining bronchial hygiene to prevent chest infection.

One longitudinal study conducted by McClaran et al. (1995) shows a 12% decline in maximum voluntary ventilation over 6 years in older trained athletes. With reduced respiratory muscle strength, and diminished ventilatory response to high demand states (Sharma and Goodwin 2006), we can expect poorer post-operative outcomes especially amongst geriatric patients.

13.4   Physiotherapy Interventions

Physiotherapists will usually assess the patient before and after surgery. The objectives of preoperative management are:
1. To establish baseline physical function
2. To assess lung function before surgery
3. To educate patient on aims of physiotherapy to optimise preoperative function
4. To educate patient on physiotherapeutic management and milestones after surgery

The objectives of post-operative management are:
1. To reassess physical/lung function post-operatively
2. To manage secretions
3. To prevent post-operative pneumonia
4. To optimise lung function post-operatively
5. To regain/optimise physical mobility

13.4.1 Bronchial Hygiene in Prevention of Post-operative Chest Complications

All surgical patients who have undergone general anaesthesia will experience some degree of sputum retention as general anaesthesia causes temporary paralysis of mucociliary action, impairing the body's natural mode of mucosal clearance. High fraction of inspired oxygen concentrations without humidification given post-operatively can also dry out the bronchial lining and further enhances mucociliary dysfunction (Denehy and van der Leur 2004). Compounding secretion retention is potential cough inhibition secondary to post-operative abdominal pain. The inability to effectively maintain bronchial hygiene can cause mucus plugging, oxygen desaturation, atelectasis and pneumonia. Physiotherapy techniques such as deep breathing exercises, supported coughing and forced expiratory techniques are used to aid removal of secretions and prevent other chest complications.

13.4.1.1 Deep Breathing Exercises

Deep breathing exercises are generally used to improve ventilation after surgery. They are also used in conjunction with forced expiratory techniques (discussed below) to aid mucociliary clearance. Also known as thoracic expansion exercises, this involves taking a deep breath, usually with an inspiratory hold of 3 s at the end. When lung volume is increased, resistance through the collateral ventilatory airways decreases and lung parenchyma are recruited, ensuring air flow behind secretions in order to aid removal of mucus (Hough 2001). Usually 3–5 deep breathing exercises are taught to aid in lung re-expansion and secretion clearance, while preventing breathlessness and fatigue.

13.4.1.2 Forced Expiratory Technique

An alternative to coughing is the forced expiratory technique (FET). This consists of 'huffing' once or twice in order to dynamically compress the airways towards the equal pressure point which is the mouth (West 2004). This technique is usually carried out following deep breathing exercises. This helps to mobilise secretions further up the airways, where a cough can be elicited to clear the secretions into the mouth for expectoration. Although a 'huff' is a forced manoeuvre, it is not a violent one and may cause less pain in patients post-abdominal surgery. Adequate analgesia should also be prescribed in order to maximise the effectiveness of a cough to clear secretions (Fig. 13.1).

13.4.1.3 Supported Coughing

Effective airway clearance depends on two factors – mucociliary clearance and an effective cough. If one of these mechanisms is disrupted, retention of secretions

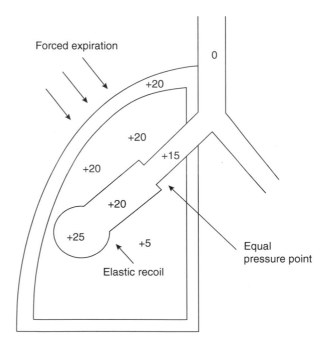

Fig. 13.1 Equal pressure point

may occur. An effective cough may be impaired by abdominal pain from the incision site. Supported coughing is one method employed by physiotherapists to reduce pain caused by coughing in the early stages of recovery. A towel is placed over the incision site and pressure applied by the patient or therapist in order to splint the wound during increased abdominal pressure associated with a cough (Fig. 13.2).

Patient education is key to patient's compliance to breathing exercises and supported cough to prevent post-operative chest complications is their understanding of their risks and how the strategies would decrease these risks.

13.4.2 To Increase Lung Volumes

Low lung volume has been shown to increase the risk of post-operative lung complications such as pneumonia and atelectasis (Dajaczman et al. 1991; Horowits et al. 1989). Abdominal distension may also exacerbate these problems.

A reduction in lung volume and flow rate with increased work of breathing, would together lead to a decrease in functional residual capacity (FRC). This may contribute to the closure of dependent airways and thereby reduce arterial oxygenation. Leblanc (1970) also noted that this effect may be accentuated in older persons.

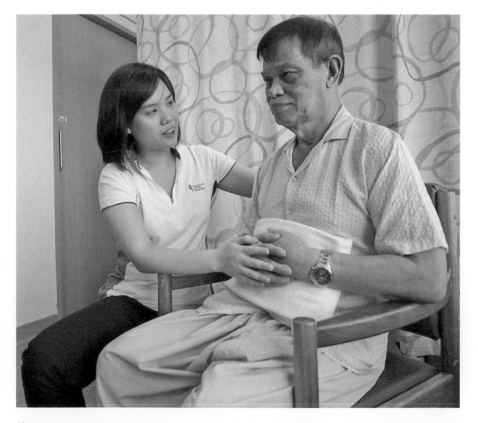

Fig. 13.2 Supported coughing

Techniques that may be used to reverse low lung volume include:
• Deep breathing with tactile facilitation
• Incentive spirometry
• Positioning
• Mobilisation/ambulation

13.4.2.1 Deep Breathing Exercises

Deep breathing exercises, also known as thoracic expansion exercises, should be taught to patients preoperatively and reinforced post-operatively. This involves tactile facilitation to the patient's lateral chest walls to increase bucket handle movement of the ribs and encourage slow, controlled inspiration. Studies show that performing hourly deep breathing exercises may reduce the risk of post-operative complications (Westerdahl et al. 2005). In addition, a 3-second inspiratory hold should be used to maintain increased transpulmonary pressure (Browning and Denehy 2007; Platell and Hall 1997) (Fig. 13.3).

13.4.2.2 Incentive Spirometry

Incentive spirometry is a common adjunct to deep breathing exercises, used especially when visual feedback is required to encourage deep breathing. More recent research has demonstrated little support of its effectiveness post-operatively (Restropo et al. 2011; Chuter et al. 1989) noted that the use of incentive spirometry failed to increase

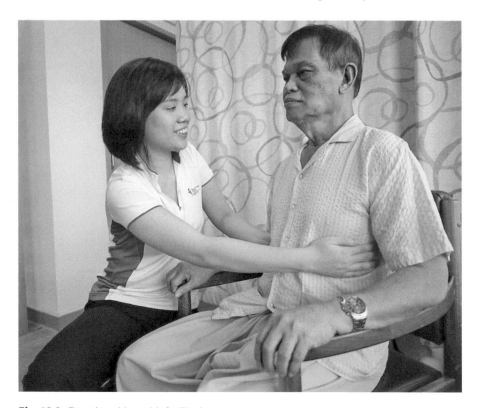

Fig. 13.3 Deep breathing with facilitation

diaphragmatic movement in post-operative patients. However, a selected group of patients who are immobile, and require visual feedback for more effective thoracic expansion exercises, may benefit from the use of an incentive spirometer (Ridley and Heinl-Green 2007).

13.4.2.3 Positioning

When positioning a patient, physiotherapists must account for the patient's current clinical presentation, laboratory test results and radiographic imaging (Dean 2007). Positioning improves V/Q matching in the lung where apices have greater initial volume and reduced compliance compared to the bases of the lungs. Conversely, lung bases are more compliant and exhibit greater volume changes during ventilation. Accordingly, the supine position has been associated with significant reductions in lung volumes and flow rates.

On the first day post-surgery, patients should be assisted to an upright position such as sitting on the edge of the bed, sitting out of bed or ambulating, depending on medical stability. The positional change from supine to upright increases functional residual capacity significantly to reverse atelectasis and positively alters lung mechanics and flow rates (Wiren et al. 1983; Mynster 1996; Nielsen et al. 2003).

13.4.2.4 Early Mobilisation

With adequate pain and nutritional management, early mobilisation post colorectal surgery has been shown to be safe and effective (Wilmore and Kehlet 2001). Functional activities such as sitting in a chair or walking are part of activities of daily living and facilitate mental well-being in addition to benefitting the respiratory system. Altered ciliary mechanics after general anaesthesia can be reversed by mobilisation/ambulation to ensure natural deep breaths are taken with movement, which can help mobilise secretions and stimulate a cough reflex.

13.4.3 Physical Reconditioning/Early Mobilisation and Conditioning of the Elderly

Very few geriatric patients advance to higher levels of physical activity after major surgery because it is often assumed that bed rest is preferable and safer. However, this perception is erroneous as bed rest has deleterious effects, especially in the elderly population.

Post-operatively, early mobilisation, facilitated with optimised pain control, can decrease the length of hospital stay, prevent functional decline and expedite functional recovery (Cruz-Jentoft et al. 2010; Browning et al. 2007). Early mobilisation of patients reduces the risk of deep venous thrombosis formation – a common complication of sudden reduction in mobility – by preventing venous stasis and pooling of blood in the lower extremities.

The spectrum of mobilisation and reconditioning spans from limb and bed mobility exercises to the practice of functional activities such as getting out of bed to sit on a chair and hallway ambulation with or without assistance. Geriatric rehabilitation also includes exercises to increase muscular endurance, muscular strength and balance.

In the acute post-operative days, when the elderly patient is feeling less able, reha-bilitation may be less vigorous, such as range of movement exercises, and simple bed or chair exercises. As the individual progresses through the acute phase, physiother-apy treatment shifts its focus towards functional factors contributing to the patient's return to premorbid status. This will include strengthening exercises such as half-squats, stairs climbing, and progressive ambulation, static and dynamic balance train-ing in both sitting and standing, and internal/external perturbation exercises, and gentle progression of cardiovascular exercises (i.e. pedal cycling, hand ergometry). By offering a holistic approach in rehabilitation of the post-surgical elderly patient, we can optimise their return to premorbid physical functional status (Fig. 13.4).

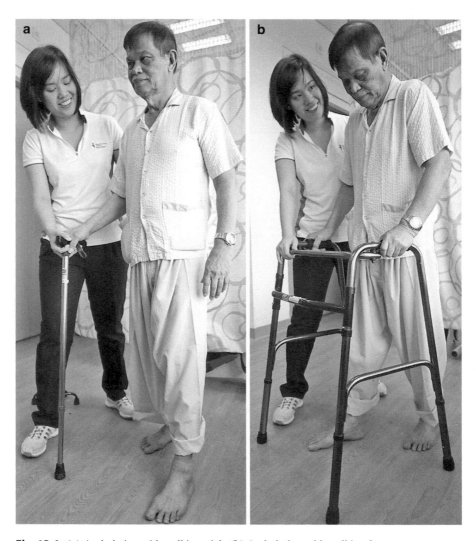

Fig. 13.4 (**a**) Ambulation with walking stick. (**b**) Ambulation with walking frame

Conclusion

By starting physiotherapy early in the geriatric population, undesirable effects of post-operative muscle weakness and atrophy can be targeted by promoting a culture of early mobility from various health-care professionals. This will be crucial, in facilitating functional recovery and a return to premorbid function.

Physiotherapy is an integral component of the holistic care of the elderly patient post-surgery. As this patient population group are more susceptible to potential physiological and physical challenges that may limit their ability to return to premorbid levels, a well and timely coordination of care within the multidisciplinary team is paramount. The physiotherapist would need to have a thorough understanding of a patient's journey from hospitalisation, through surgery, to discharge, as well as appreciate the surgical considerations that may limit a patient's physical outcome.

Other issues such as optimising pain management prior to therapy sessions and early planning of discharge are some of the many considerations that a physiotherapist will need to collaborate on with the other members of the transdisciplinary team to ensure an all-rounded supportive holistic care for the patient.

References

Berend N (2005) Normal ageing of the lung: implications for diagnosis and monitoring asthma in older people. Med J Aust 183:S28–S29

Browning L, Denehy L, Scholes RL (2007) The quantity of early upright mobilisation performed following upper abdominal surgery is low: an observational study. Aust J Physiother 53:47–52

Chuter TA, Weissman C, Starker PM et al (1989) Effect of incentive spirometry on diaphragmatic function after surgery. Surgery 105; 4:488–493

Craig DB (1981) Postoperative recovery of pulmonary function. Anaesthesia and Analgesia 60:46–52

Cruz-Jentoft AJ, Landi F, Topinková E et al (2010) Understanding sarcopenia as a geriatric syndrome. Curr Opin Clin Nutr Metab Care 13(1):1–7

Dajaczman E, Gordon A, Kreisman H et al (1991) Long term post thoracotomy pain. Chest 99:270–274

Dean E (2007) Effects of positioning and mobilization. In: Pryor JA, Prasad SA (eds) Physiotherapy for respiratory and cardiac problems in adults and paediatrics, 3rd edn. Churchill Livingstone, Edinburgh

Denehy L, van der Leur J (2004) Postoperative mucus clearance. In: Rubins B, van der Schans C (eds) Therapy for mucus-clearance disorders. Marcel Dekker, New York

Denehy L (2008) Surgery for Adults. In: Pryor JA, Prasad SA (eds) Physiotehrapy for respiratory and cardiac problems in adults and paediatrics, 4th Ed, Churchill Livingstone, Edinburgh

Durrant V, Moore K (2004) Early mobilisation of post-surgical patients. ACPRC J 36:32–36

Horowits MD, Ancalmo N, Ochsner JL (1989) Thoracotomy through auscultatory triangle. Ann Thorac Surg 47:782–783

Hough A (2001) Physiotherapy to increase lung volume. In: Hough A (ed) Physiotherapy in respiratory care, 3rd edn. Nelson Thornes Ltd, Cheltenham

Inouye SK, Studenski S, Tinetti ME et al (2007) Geriatric syndromes: clinical, research, and policy implications of a core geriatric concept. J Am Geriatr Soc 55:780–791

Leblanc P, Ruff F, Milic-Emili (1970) Effects of age and body. Position on airway closure in man. Journal of Applied Physiology 28:448–451

McClaran SR, Babcock Ma, Pegelow DF et al (1995) Longitudinal effects of aging on lung function at rest and exercise in healthy active at elderly adults. Journal of Applied Physiology 78; 5:1957–1968

Mynster T (1996) The effect of posture on late postoperative oxygenation. Anaesthesia 51:225–227

Nielsen KG, Holte K, Kehlet H (2003) Effects of posture on postoperative pulmonary function. Acta Anaesthesiol Scand 47:1270–1277

Platell C, Hall JC (1997) Atelectasis after abdominal surgery. Journal of American College of Surgeons 185:584–592

Restropo RD, Wettstein R, Wittrebel L (2011) AARC Clinical Practice Guideline: Incentive Spirometry. Respiratory Care 56; 10:1600–1604

Ridley S, Heinl-Green A (2007) Surgery for adults. In: Pryor JA, Prasad SA (eds) Physiotherapy for respiratory and cardiac problems in adults and paediatrics, 3rd edn. Churchill Livingstone, Edinburgh

Sharma G, Goodwin J (2006) Effect of ageing on respiratory system physiology and immunology. Clin Interv Aging 1(3):253–260

Van Craen K, Braes T, Wellens N et al (2010) The effectiveness of inpatient geriatric evaluation and management units: a systematic review and meta-analysis. J Am Geriatr Soc 58:83–92

West JB (2004) Respiratory physiology – the essentials, 7th edn. Williams and Wilkins, Baltimore

Westerdahl E, Lindmark B, Eriksson T et al (2005) Deep breathing exercises reduce atelectasis and improve pulmonary function after coronary artery bypass surgery. Chest 128:3482–3488

Wilmore DW, Kehlet H (2001) Management of patients in fast track surgery. Br Med J 322:473–476

Wiren JE, Lindell SE, Hellekant C (1983) Pre- and postoperative lung function in sitting and supine position related to postoperative chest X-ray abnormalities and arterial hypoxaemia. Clin Physiol 3:257–266

Perioperative Urinary Problems in Older Surgical Patients

14

Terence Tang

Take Home Pearls

- Contributors of urinary symptoms and incontinence in older adults, apart from bladder dysfunction, include functional causes such as mobility, cognition, and environmental barriers.
- Bladder dysfunction in the perioperative period is usually caused by multiple reasons ranging from predisposing causes, surgical injury, and various perioperative complications.
- A holistic approach and assessment is needed to identify and address these urinary issues for these older surgical patients.
- The approach is divided into storage symptoms (typified by urinary incontinence) and voiding symptoms (typified by retention of urine).

14.1   Introduction

With the rising prevalence of colonic malignancies in the population, coupled with an aging society, it is not uncommon to encounter the need to evaluate older adults undergoing colorectal surgery. Despite improvement in colorectal surgical techniques, since its inception 100 years ago (Lange et al. 2009), morbidities from these surgical procedures are prevalent and can be equally disabling. Bladder dysfunction following earlier pelvic colorectal procedures reached 50% with abdominoperineal resections and up to 25% in low anterior resections (Mannaerts et al. 2001).

T. Tang
Department of Geriatric Medicine,
Khoo Teck Puat Hospital, Alexandra Health, Singapore, Singapore
e-mail: tang.terence.ey@alexandrahealth.com.sg

K.-Y. Tan (ed.), *Colorectal Cancer in the Elderly*,
DOI 10.1007/978-3-642-29883-7_14, © Springer-Verlag Berlin Heidelberg 2013

These figures are not surprising as the primary goal of surgical resection is to bring about oncologic cure and this is achieved through wide resections with clear margins. The cost of cure invariably hinges between surgical clearance and the expense of surrounding tissues, in particular, the autonomic innervations of the pelvic viscera and the anal sphincters. The end result can be significant urogenital morbidity with urinary and fecal incontinence. Increased awareness of the pelvic nerves and nerve preservation surgical techniques have improved overall results. In this section, we examine the issues of urinary control in older adults undergoing colorectal surgery.

14.2 Physiology of Voiding

The bladder has two basic functions. It serves to *hold* urine as the kidneys are producing it and to *empty* it when it is full, at a convenient time and place. The bladder is essentially an expansible bag of smooth muscles, which undergoes the micturition cycle comprising of the filling phase and the voiding (emptying) phase. The normal micturition cycle requires the complex coordination of the frontal cortex, hypothalamus, brainstem, as well as the spinal centers. This complex process involves the interactions between conscious and unconscious control mediated via the somatic and autonomic innervations. It is generally agreed that there are three major groups of nerves involved in normal urinary function (Kevorkian 2004). These are particularly at risk during pelvic dissections.

14.2.1 Parasympathetic Innervations

The pelvic splanchnic nerves provide the parasympathetic (S2–S4) innervations to the pelvic organs. The nerves emerge from the sacrum and run ventrally and laterally to join the sympathetic nerves forming the inferior hypogastric complex and anteriorly to Denovilliers fascia as well. The parasympathetic nerves serve to effect detrusor contractions through the release of acetylcholine at the neuromuscular junction and thus voiding. These nerves also contain sensory afferents, which carry sensations of bladder filling. Damage to these nerves can result in an insensate bladder and detrusor under activity.

14.2.2 Sympathetic Innervations

The superior hypogastric plexuses (L3–S1) run parallel with the ureters and join the inferior hypogastric complex in the pelvis. The sympathetic component of the autonomic nervous system serves to relax the detrusor muscles and simultaneous contraction of the trigone and bladder neck through the release of norepinephrine on beta-adrenoceptors. These allow the bladder to relax, fill, and hold urine. Damage will result in an incompetent bladder neck with urinary incontinence.

14.2.3 Somatic Sensorimotor Innervations

The pudendal nerve arises from the sacral outflow tract (S2–S4). This is the somatic component which runs through the Alcock's canal and follows the perineal artery into the superficial pouch to supply the ischiocavernosus, bulbospongiosus, and transverse perinei muscles, as well as the levator ani and striated urethral sphincter. Some branches continue anteriorly to supply sensation to the posterior scrotum and perineum. Damage to the pudendal nerve results in the loss of voluntary contraction of the external striated urethral sphincter and hence urinary incontinence (Delacroix and Winters 2010; Kevorkian 2004).

Finally, it must be understood that the act of voiding is a complex human activity that involves many physiological processes taking the person from awareness of a full bladder, the concept of a washroom as an appropriate place for voiding, the ability to search and ambulate, the dexterity of one's hands to unclothe and then to effect the voiding. A breakdown in any of these processes will result in urinary incontinence. The predisposition of frailty, multiple comorbidities, medications, and the impact of the surgical process must be taken into account when assessing the incontinent elderly in the perioperative period.

14.3   Perioperative Assessment of Urinary Function

The older patient is already predisposed to urinary problems prior to any surgical procedures. Urinary symptoms and incontinence occur in 14–25% of community-dwelling older persons, one third of persons in acute care hospitals and in more than 50% of those in nursing homes (Diokno 2001; Espino et al. 2003; Maggi et al. 2001). Older persons who are prone are likely to be physically or cognitively frail and need assistance in their activities of daily living. These predispositions are added upon by the stress of the colorectal disease, the hospitalization, the use of various anesthetic and analgesic medications, as well as the surgical procedures.

It is important to first determine the onset of lower urinary tract symptoms, bearing in mind that these can occur prior to the surgery. These symptoms can be largely classified into two broad categories (Morley 2004):

14.3.1 Voiding Symptoms

Symptoms associated with difficulty in emptying the bladder. These include hesitancy, intermittency, slow or weak stream, terminal dribbling, straining, incomplete voiding, or the complete inability to void.

14.3.2 Storage Symptoms

Symptoms associated with difficulty in holding the bladder. These include urgency, frequency, stress symptoms (leakage with increased intra-abdominal pressure, e.g., coughing, laughing, straining), and urinary incontinence.

Once the above symptoms are established, the approach can be as follows. The causes of these symptoms can be largely divided into three categories: precipitating, functional, and established causes. Although, it is also important to note that the causes of the urinary symptoms are often multifactorial in nature.

14.3.3 Precipitating Causes

These are usually transient and precipitate a crisis of urinary incontinence or acute retention of urine. Common causes include:
- Delirium
- Urinary tract infection
- Atrophic vaginitis
- Pain
- Prolonged recumbrancy
- Decreased or impaired mobility
- Pharmacological agents such as narcotic analgesia (e.g., morphine, tramadol)
- Psychological states of anxiety and depression
- Hyperglycemia and hypercalcemia
- Constipation

14.3.4 Functional Causes

There are occasions in which the urinary symptoms arise from causes not otherwise related to the control of the bladder. These include physical barriers such as restraints or communication barriers between the patient and the health-care workers. Other causes include the inability to get to the toilet or the loss of ability of recognizing the need to void in the toilet (e.g., dementia and delirium) (Morley 2004).

14.3.5 Established Causes

These refer to causes that are deep seated and may not be easily reversible. These can arise from the surgery itself or are already present prior to the surgery. Common causes include:

For voiding symptoms:
- Bladder outlet obstruction such as BPH, urethral strictures, and prolapsed pelvic organ
- Prolonged bladder distension with consequent detrusor under activity (e.g., prolonged catheter obstruction or constipation)
- Diabetic autonomic neuropathy
- Spinal cord compression (e.g., degenerative spine disease, spinal metastases)
- Pelvic surgical injury to the autonomic innervations

For storage symptoms:
- Underlying overactive bladder syndrome
- Preexisting pelvic floor muscle weakness
- Surgical injury and alteration of pelvic floor anatomy and function
- Pelvic surgical injury to the autonomic innervations

Most of the precipitating and functional causes can be easily excluded at the bedside with a focused history, review of the medications, and a directed physical examination (Kevorkian 2004). The physical examination should include the following:

- Abdominal examination with a rectal examination and in women, a pelvic examination
- Neurologic examination of the lower limbs
- Brief mental state examination
- Brief assessment of the functional and mobility state

The physical examination can be further augmented by various quick bedside investigations:

- Bladder scan for post void residual urinary volume to determine urinary retention
- Urine dipstick for leucocytes and blood to suggest urinary tract infection
- Capillary blood glucose level to establish hyperglycemia

The above evaluation would be sufficient in most cases. However, in selected patients or patients who fail initial therapeutic trials, advanced investigations such as imaging studies of the spine and pelvic organs, cystoscopy, as well as uroflowmetry and pressure-flow urodynamic studies may be required.

14.4 Management

The perioperative management of the elderly patients undergoing colorectal surgery is individualized and multidimensional in nature. It requires a transdisciplinary team comprising of the surgeon, anesthetist, geriatrician, nursing, their team of therapists, social workers, dietitian, and the involvement of the patient and family members (Tan et al. 2011). Focus on patients' bladder and bowel control should begin at the preoperative period and to compare that to the postoperative state.

The successful removal of catheter postoperatively is not synonymous with the return of normal bladder function. Urinary symptoms especially voiding symptoms with sustained increase in residual urine volumes can often be found in patients undergoing low anterior or abdominoperineal resection (Chaudhri et al. 2006). Patients with overt symptoms of urinary retention after colorectal surgery need to be quickly decompressed, while the clinical significance of moderately elevated residual urine (100–200 mls) remains controversial. These patients should be followed closely for the development of urinary retention subsequently.

Bladder decompression can be done via inserting an indwelling catheter (e.g., size 14–18 gauge French Foley's catheter) to allow temporary evacuation of the residual urine. Probable precipitants of bladder outlet obstruction should be identified and removed. Predisposing causes such as BPH must also be addressed, and a trial with α-adrenergic antagonists may be necessary. The patients should also be actively encouraged to get out of bed and start ambulating. Trials regarding the optimal timing of removal of catheter showed conflicting results. The bladder is generally allowed to "rest" for about a week or two before a trial of removal of the catheter (Delacroix and Winters 2010). Patients who fail to recover after the initial trial can be given an extended period of recovery. They will, however, require plans for prolonged interim urethral catheterization.

Longer-term catheterization can be done via two methods. Patients can either be sent home with an indwelling urinary catheter and bag or are trained to perform the clean intermittent catheterization (CIC). CIC is performed with a 12–14 French low friction catheter every 4–6 h. Motivated caregivers can also be trained to assist or perform the CIC for these patients. The patients are asked to void and empty their bladders before CIC is performed. The amount of residual volume is then charted, and its trend is especially helpful in determining the recovery of the detrusor muscles. CIC can be stopped when volumes reach below 200 mls. For patients who remain unable to void, further evaluation with pressure-flow urodynamic studies and cystoscopy may be necessary at approximately 2–3 months postoperatively.

Conversely, patients can also experience storage symptoms and urinary incontinence in the postoperative setting. These patients may represent extensive bladder injury from their procedure or as a result of neurogenic alteration. Nonetheless, common precipitating causes and predisposing conditions must be identified and mitigated. The patient is reassured and incontinence must be temporarily contained with adsorbent pads or continence appliances such as the urinal or bedside commode.

In the absence of precipitating causes, troublesome symptoms such as urgency can be alleviated with the use of anticholinergic medications. Drugs such as oxybutynin, tolterodine, trospium chloride, solifenacin, and darifenacin can be used for the management of urinary urgency. It is important to note that the adverse effects of these drugs must be monitored with dose escalation (MacDiarmid 2003). Adverse effects include confusion, blurring of vision, constipation, dry mouth, urinary retention, and the precipitation of closed angle glaucoma. Only in refractory symptoms of detrusor overactivity, patients are offered intra-vesicle botulinum toxin injections and the use of neuromodulation (Delacroix and Winters 2010).

In the subgroup who present with features of stress incontinence and bladder neck incompetence, the causes are usually attributed to autonomic or somatic denervation, surgical disruption to the pelvic anatomy, or predisposing pelvic floor weakness. A trial of pelvic exercise can offer some improvement over the control of the bladder. In more severe cases with intractable urinary leakage, various bladder neck sling operations can be offered in women. For more severe degrees of incontinence in men, the artificial urinary sphincter is an option (Webster et al. 1992).

14.5   Summary

Bladder dysfunction after pelvic colorectal surgery is relatively common. The prevalence is high in older surgical techniques but has improved with newer surgical techniques (Chessin and Guillem 2005). Nonetheless, the predisposition in older patients to bladder dysfunction will be amplified during the perioperative period given the stressors of hospitalization, anesthesia, and surgery. With the proper approach, the causes of urinary problems in the perioperative period, though multifactorial in nature, can be easily identified and reversed. The commonest etiology of longer-term urinary retention is from autonomic disruption from the surgical procedures. Majority of these cases will resolve within the first 6 months, usually with no long-term sequelae (Delacroix and Winters 2010). However, these patients must be monitored and managed to prevent secondary bladder damage from prolonged over-distension, infection, and possibly hydronephrosis and renal failure. Treatment and follow-up are highly individualized based on clinical and investigational findings. The transdisciplinary team must take into account patient expectations, abilities, and the family support with the aim of the more than just oncologic cure but eventual return to function in the community.

References

Chaudhri S, Maruthachalam K, Kaiser A, Robson W, Pickard RS, Horgan AF (2006) Successful voiding after trial without catheter is not synonymous with recovery of bladder function after colorectal surgery. Dis Colon Rectum 49(7):1066–1070

Chessin DB, Guillem JG (2005) Abdominoperineal resection for rectal cancer: historic perspective and current issues. Surg Oncol Clin N Am 14(3):569–586, vii

Delacroix SE Jr, Winters JC (2010) Voiding dysfunction after pelvic colorectal surgery. Clin Colon Rectal Surg 23(2):119–127

Diokno AC (2001) Epidemiology of urinary incontinence. J Gerontol A Biol Sci Med Sci 56A:M3–M4

Espino DV, Palmer RF, Miles TP, Mouton CP, Lichtenstein MJ, Markides KP (2003) Prevalence and severity of urinary incontinence in elderly Mexican-American women. J Am Geriatr Soc 51:1580–1586

Kevorkian R (2004) Physiology of incontinence. Clin Geriatr Med 20:409–425

Lange MM, Rutten HJ, van de Velde CJ (2009) One hundred years of curative surgery for rectal cancer: 1908–2008. Eur J Surg Oncol 35(5):456–463

MacDiarmid SA (2003) Overactive bladder: improving the efficacy of anticholinergics by dose escalation. Curr Urol Rep 4(6):446–451

Maggi S, Minicuci N, Langlois J, Pavan M, Enzi G, Crepaldi G (2001) Prevalence rate of urinary incontinence in community-dwelling elderly individuals: the Veneto study. J Gerontol A Biol Sci Med Sci 56A:M14–M18

Mannaerts GH, Schijven MP, Hendrikx A, Martijn H, Rutten HJ, Wiggers T (2001) Urologic and sexual morbidity following multimodality treatment for locally advanced primary and locally recurrent rectal cancer. Eur J Surg Oncol 27(3):265–272

Morley JE (2004) Urinary incontinence and the community-dwelling elder: a practical approach to diagnosis and management for the primary care geriatrician. Clin Geriatr Med 20:427–435

Tan KY, Tan P, Tan L (2011) A collaborative transdisciplinary "geriatric surgery service" ensures consistent successful outcomes in elderly colorectal surgery patients. World J Surg 35(7):1608–1614

Webster GD, Perez LM, Khoury JM, Timmons SL (1992) Management of type III stress urinary incontinence using artificial urinary sphincter. Urology 39(6):499–503

Adjuvant Chemotherapy for Senior Patients After Resection of Colon Cancer

15

Simon Yew-Kuang Ong

Take Home Pearls

- Elderly patients with colorectal cancer will continue to grow significantly in numbers, importance, and relevance.
- After surgery, they often fail to receive the standard of care, which in part is due to physician's perception that they will not benefit from adjuvant chemotherapy.
- Carefully selected elderly patients do benefit from and tolerate adjuvant chemotherapy like their younger counterparts.
- A multidimensional screening tool such as the comprehensive geriatric assessment and a multidisciplinary approach is helpful in selecting and individualizing care for the elderly cancer patients.
- Elderly-specific trials and study endpoints are needed to address the unanswered questions in this subpopulation of cancer patients.

15.1   Introduction

Colorectal cancer is a leading cancer in most developed countries. It predominantly affects older people, and its incidence increases with increasing age. Locally, it is the most frequent cancer overall, and its incidence rises sharply at the age 65 or greater (Seow et al. 2004). This vulnerable segment of the population is increasing among the developed nations (Yancik 2005; Yancik and Ries 2004). In a survey of 21 major countries, Singapore was estimated to have the second highest percentage

S.Y.-K. Ong
Department of Medical Oncology, National Cancer Center, Singapore
e-mail: dmooyk@nccs.com.sg

K.-Y. Tan (ed.), *Colorectal Cancer in the Elderly*,
DOI 10.1007/978-3-642-29883-7_15, © Springer-Verlag Berlin Heidelberg 2013

increase of the elderly population (≥60 years) between 1985 and 2025. Even more worrying will be the projected eightfold increase in the very old (≥75 years) by 2020 (Choo et al. 1990, 1991). This makes colorectal cancer in the older patient a socially and epidemiologically important cancer locally, and its relevance can only grow as the number of older people increases.

Older people with cancer also pose special challenges to the cancer physician. Older patients are often perceived to benefit less from cancer treatment because of limited life expectancy and competing causes of mortality. They are also perceived to experience greater toxicity because of diminished organ reserves and multiple comorbidities. Physicians often perceive that older people are less willing to undergo toxic chemotherapy. Older people may face greater socioeconomic barriers to receiving chemotherapy.

This review will explore the pattern of utilization, preferences, benefits, and toxicity associated with adjuvant chemotherapy in the elderly patient with stage III colon cancer. Additionally, this review will also examine the potential implications of treatment dose reduction and early termination, role of adjuvant chemotherapy for stage II disease, and which patients to treat and what regimen to use. It is beyond the scope of this review to encompass the role of radiotherapy in the elderly patient with rectal cancer.

15.2 What Is the Standard of Care for Patients with Resected Stage III Colon Cancer?

15.2.1 Fluoropyrimidine-Based Adjuvant Therapy

Adjuvant chemotherapy after curative resection of stage III colon cancer is well established. After the Intergroup Trial INT-0035 first reported a significant reduction in the risk of death with adjuvant 5-fluorouracil/levamisole in patients with stage III colon cancer (Moertel et al. 1990), the NIH (National Institutes of Health) recommended that 5-fluorouracil/levamisole for 1 year should be prescribed routinely for patients in this setting (NIH Consensus Conference 1990). Five years later, the IMPACT (International Multicenter Pooled Analysis of B2 Colon Cancer Trials) investigators reported that 5-fluorouracil/leucovorin for 6 months is an effective, well-tolerated, and shorter adjuvant regimen for colon cancer (Efficacy of adjuvant fluorouracil and folinic acid in colon cancer. IMPACT investigators 1995). Subsequently, it was shown that the oral fluoropyrimidines, namely, capecitabine and UFT (tegafur/uracil), could be used as an equivalent alternative to intravenous 5-fluorouracil (Twelves et al. 2005a; Lembersky et al. 2006). The various fluoropyrimidine-based adjuvant regimens discussed so far are regarded as single-agent regimens because levamisole and leucovorin are considered as treatment modulators.

15.2.2 Oxaliplatin-Based Adjuvant Therapy

More recently, the landmark MOSAIC (Multicenter International Study of Oxaliplatin/5-Fluorouracil/Leucovorin in the Adjuvant Treatment of Colon Cancer) study demonstrated for the first time that the use of a combination regimen, adding oxaliplatin to infusion 5-fluorouracil/leucovorin (FOLFOX), improves the adjuvant treatment of colon cancer compared to 5-fluorouracil/leucovorin alone. Based on the initial results of this study and the updated report at 6 years of follow-up, FOLFOX is currently firmly accepted as the standard of care in patients after resection for stage III colon cancer (Andre et al. 2004, 2009). The results of NSABP (National Surgical Adjuvant Breast and Bowel Project) C07 study validate the benefits of adding oxaliplatin to 5-fluorouracil in stage II and III colon cancer (Kuebler et al. 2007). Other investigators are now studying the role of substituting the intravenous 5-fluorouracil with oral capecitabine for combining with oxaliplatin. Early data from the NO16968 study suggests that XELOX (capecitabine/oxaliplatin or CAPOX) is superior to 5-fluorouracil/leucovorin for disease-free survival (Haller et al. 2010).

15.2.3 Irinotecan-Based Adjuvant Therapy

Although FOLFIRI (irinotecan plus 5-fluorouracil/leucovorin) is accepted as an equally active regimen compared to FOLFOX in the metastatic setting, irinotecan-based regimens have failed to benefit patients who were treated in the adjuvant setting. Three large phase III trials, one US and two European studies, comparing irinotecan/5-fluorouracil/leucovorin with 5-fluorouracil/leucovorin did not result in any survival benefit (Saltz et al. 2007; Van Cutsem et al. 2009; Ychou et al. 2009). Importantly, these trials demonstrate that advances in the treatment of metastatic disease do not necessarily translate into advances in the curative setting.

15.2.4 Adjuvant Targeted Therapy

Meanwhile, two monoclonal antibodies, bevacizumab and cetuximab, which have demonstrated activity in advanced colorectal cancer therapy, are now being evaluated in large randomized studies in the adjuvant setting. Results from the NSABP C08 study did not show any benefit when bevacizumab for 1 year was added to FOLFOX (Allegra et al. 2011). A major pan-European collaboration (PETACC-8) exploring cetuximab as adjuvant therapy in stage III colon cancer is ongoing.

15.2.5 NCCN Guidelines

For stage III colon cancer, the NCCN (National Comprehensive Cancer Network) panel recommends FOLFOX as the preferred option and capecitabine/oxaliplatin as an alternative; single-agent capecitabine or 5-fluorouracil/leucovorin in patients felt to be inappropriate for oxaliplatin therapy. The panel does not recommend the use of cetuximab, bevacizumab, or irinotecan in adjuvant therapy for nonmetastatic colon cancer (NCCN Clinical Practice Guidelines in Oncology [NCCN Guidelines] 2011).

15.3   Are Senior Cancer Patients Prescribed the Standard of Care?

15.3.1 Fewer Older Patients Receive Adjuvant Chemotherapy

The use of adjuvant chemotherapy decreases dramatically with increasing age. A population-based analysis of colon cancer patient data from the SEER (National Cancer Institute's Surveillance, Epidemiology, and End Results) database was carried out looking for the association of 5-fluorouracil chemotherapy and survival in older patients (Sundararajan et al. 2002). There were 4,768 patients aged ≥65 who were diagnosed with stage III colon cancer from 1992 to 1996. This survey reported that 52% of the patients received adjuvant chemotherapy. However, only 11% of the older patients (mean age, 87) received treatment compared to 83% in the younger group (mean, 69 years). This trend of decrease in usage of chemotherapy with advancing age was seen even in patients without any major comorbidity (Quipourt et al. 2011; Schrag et al. 2001). Results from several other analyses, which also examined patients' data from the SEER database, showed the same decrease in utilization of adjuvant therapy among the older patients (Jessup et al. 2005; Kahn et al. 2010; Schrag et al. 2001).

15.3.2 Older Patients Are Prescribed Less Toxic Regimens

Physicians were more likely to use less toxic regimens with increasing age. Investigators from Dana-Farber/Harvard Cancer Center examined the treatment records from 2,560 patients treated at 122 medical oncology centers across 35 US states to determine the pattern and duration of use of adjuvant chemotherapy in resected stage II and III colon cancer patients (Abrams et al. 2011). Between 2004 and 2010, patients received capecitabine, 5-fluorouracil, CAPOX, or FOLFOX. This study recorded that 86% of patients aged <60 received FOLFOX or CAPOX for their adjuvant treatment compared to only 42% in patients aged ≥80. A smaller observational CanCORS (Cancer Care Outcomes Research and Surveillance) study analyzed care delivered to patients in the USA to determine the use and outcomes of adjuvant chemotherapy in older patients (≥70 years) with stage III colon cancer (Kahn et al. 2010). Among the patients treated with adjuvant chemotherapy, 14% of the older patients versus 44% of the young patients received an oxaliplatin-based therapy. Similarly, among the 252 patients with stage III colon cancer treated at four Australian hospitals, 20% of the patients older than 70 years of age received adjuvant FOLFOX compared to >90% in younger patients aged <60 (Ananda et al. 2008).

15.3.3 Fewer Older Patients Complete Adjuvant Therapy

Older patients are more likely to discontinue their treatment early. The two US studies that reported a decreased use of oxaliplatin in older patients also observed that premature termination of adjuvant chemotherapy was more likely in this group of patients. In the larger Dana-Farber/Harvard study, 30% of patients stopped their adjuvant chemotherapy after less than 3 months with age and use of oxaliplatin associated with early discontinuation of treatment (Abrams et al. 2011). In the CanCORS study, 40% of the older patients (≥65 years) terminated treatment by 150 days compared to 25% of patients in the younger age group (Kahn et al. 2010). Another large population-based study based on the SEER database specifically tried to determine the factors associated with initiation and completion of adjuvant chemotherapy for stage III colon cancer (Dobie et al. 2006). Age was a statistically significant predictor of chemotherapy completion – the likelihood of completing treatment decreased with age for those older than 75 years.

15.3.4 Physicians Less Likely to Recommend Adjuvant Therapy for Older Patients

Physicians are more conservative when recommending adjuvant chemotherapy in older patients especially when accompanied by comorbid illness. In a large national survey of cancer surgeons and medical oncologists caring for patients with colorectal cancer, it was found that the physician's recommendations varied substantially by patient age and severity of comorbidity (Keating et al. 2008). Nearly all the cancer physicians (98%) would be very likely to recommend adjuvant chemotherapy for a fit and young person, whereas most (92%) would be very or somewhat unlikely to recommend the same treatment for the old and unfit.

15.3.5 Fewer Older Patients Accept Recommendation for Treatment

Older patients are more likely to decline chemotherapy. Data from Australia suggests that patients aged ≥70 with stage III colon cancer are more likely to decline treatment against physician's advice compared to their younger counterparts – 11% versus 1.4% (Ananda et al. 2008). A study of 628 women with recently diagnosed colorectal or breast cancer was conducted by telephone to evaluate the patient's perspective of selecting cancer treatments. Older women were less likely to be offered adjuvant treatments, but they were also more likely to reject these treatments when recommended (Newcomb and Carbone 1993). When 244 cancer patients were asked to make hypothetical decisions based on four vignettes, older patients were as likely as their younger counterparts to agree to chemotherapy (Yellen et al. 1994). However, they were only willing to accept a more toxic regimen over a less toxic one provided there was a greater survival advantage. A prospective cohort study that examined the effect of age on decisions to withhold life-sustaining therapies found that older age was associated with less willingness to accept aggressive therapies such as ventilator support, surgery, or dialysis (Hamel et al. 1999). One reason for this trend could be the preference of quality of life over length of life among the older patients (Fried et al. 2002; Meropol et al. 2008).

164
S.Y.-K. Ong

15.4 Do Senior Cancer Patients Benefit from Adjuvant Chemotherapy?

There is a lack of direct evidence showing benefit of adjuvant chemotherapy in the older patients from randomized controlled studies. There is underrepresentation of older patients (≥65 years) in clinical cancer trials (Hutchins et al. 1999). Moreover, it is likely that the older patients who are successfully enrolled into clinical trials tend to be fitter than their peers. Due to the lack of good phase III data in this area, most of the evidence supporting the use of adjuvant therapy in the older patients is derived from subset analyses, secondary analyses of pooled data, or population-based analyses. Of these, the data derived from population-based studies may represent the best way to evaluate improvements in the care of the elderly colon cancer patient. The author will review the evidence of treatment benefit in older patients who have been treated with fluoropyrimidine-based and oxaliplatin-based adjuvant therapy. Although there is comparatively more evidence (phase IIs, phase IIIs, and pooled analyses) in the literature regarding treatment benefit in the elderly patients in the metastatic setting, this data will not be discussed here (Aparicio et al. 2003; Comella et al. 2005; de Gramont et al. 2000; Feliu et al. 2005, 2006; Folprecht et al. 2004; Goldberg et al. 2006; Rosati et al. 2005; Tabah-Fisch et al. 2002). The three negative irinotecan-based adjuvant studies underscore the dangers of extrapolating benefit in one setting to another (Saltz et al. 2007; van Cutsem et al. 2009; Ychou et al. 2009). Finally, this section will also review briefly whether older people live long enough to benefit from the adjuvant therapy.

15.4.1 Fluoropyrimidine-Based Adjuvant Therapy

The X-ACT trial is a phase III study involving 1,987 patients with stage III colon cancer randomized to adjuvant oral capecitabine or bolus 5-fluorouracil/leucovorin (Twelves et al. 2011). After a median of 6.9 years of follow-up, the investigators report the final results with a subset analysis by age. This updated report confirms that oral capecitabine had at least equivalent efficacy compared to 5-fluorouracil/leucovorin, which was maintained at 5 years and across all subgroups including patients aged ≥70.

A pooled analysis of seven phase III trials involving 3,351 patients with stage II/III colon cancer was performed (Sargent et al. 2001). This analysis involved the largest pooled data of patients comparing adjuvant chemotherapy (bolus 5-fluorouracil/leucovorin or levamisole) with no adjuvant therapy specifically evaluating whether older patients benefited from adjuvant treatment. Patients were grouped into four age categories: those ≤50, those from 51–60, those 61–70, and those >70. The analysis revealed that patients who received adjuvant chemotherapy experienced a significant positive survival benefit – 71% versus 64%. The improved overall survival was similar across all age groups. However, the survival curves for patients older than 70 tend to converge slightly over time. This is probably due to deaths from noncancer causes. The investigators concluded that selected elderly patients with colon cancer could achieve the same benefit from fluorouracil-based adjuvant therapy as their younger counterparts. Using the same pooled data set, the same group of investigators performed another analysis to examine the magnitude of adjuvant therapy benefit across various specific subsets such as age, sex, nodal status, T stage, grade, and location (Gill et al. 2004). They concluded that patients with high-risk resected colon cancer benefited from fluorouracil-based therapy across all subsets including age.

Several population-based analyses showed that elderly patients who received adjuvant chemotherapy had a higher probability of survival than patients who did not. Two earlier analyses based on the SEER database between 1992 and 1996 showed that adjuvant 5-fluorouracil therapy was associated with reduced mortality in the older patients (Sundararajan et al. 2002; Iwashyna and Lamont 2002). This reduced mortality was comparable with that observed in randomized controlled studies among younger patients. In one of the studies, the investigators evaluated whether the effectiveness of treatment varied with age among the elderly (Iwashyna and Lamont 2002). They found that the magnitude of benefit did not vary with age. An even larger but later analysis of the SEER database from 1997 to 2002 again showed that adjuvant chemotherapy increased survival in treated elderly patients (Zuckerman et al. 2009). However, the survival benefit appeared to decrease with increasing age: 14% when aged 70–74 compared with 8% when aged 80–84. Prospective data from 85,937 patients with stage III colon cancer from 560 hospital cancer registries were entered into the National Cancer Data Base between 1990 and 2002 (Jessup et al. 2005). Analysis showed that adjuvant chemotherapy was associated with an increase in 5-year survival by 16% and that elderly patients have the same benefit as younger patients.

The data is very consistent in showing that elderly patients can and do derive survival benefit from adjuvant fluoropyrimidine therapy. Most of the evidence indicates that the magnitude of this benefit is no different from that observed in the younger patients but at least one population-based analysis suggested that it diminished with increasing patient's age.

15.4.2 Oxaliplatin-Based Adjuvant Therapy

A pivotal phase III study (NO16968) randomized 1,886 patients with stage III colon cancer to adjuvant XELOX (CAPOX) or bolus 5-fluorouracil/leucovorin (Haller et al. 2010). Patients treated with XELOX experienced a superior 3-year disease-free survival compared to 5-fluorouracil/leucovorin – 71% versus 67%. Further analysis of the 3-year disease-free survival in patients aged <70 and those ≥70 did not show a difference in advantage.

In contrast, a subgroup analysis of a similarly designed phase III study reported contradicting findings in the elderly subset. In the MOSAIC study, FOLFOX was employed in the experimental arm instead of XELOX (Andre et al. 2004). It was this pivotal study that first established the role of FOLFOX as the standard of care in adjuvant colon cancer therapy. A subgroup analysis of elderly patients aged ≥70 in this trial was performed to determine the clinical characteristics and outcome of adjuvant treatment in older patients (Tournigand et al. 2010). In this study, the investigators found that the disease-free survival benefit of FOLFOX could be of less magnitude than in younger patients.

A pooled analysis from the ACCENT (Adjuvant Colon Cancer End Point) trial using data from six randomized controlled studies sought to determine the impact of age on treatment outcomes with the newer adjuvant options (Jackson McCleary et al. 2009). The six randomized controlled studies compared irinotecan-based, oxaliplatin-based, and oral fluoropyrimidine adjuvant therapies with bolus 5-fluorouracil in stage II and III colon cancer. This analysis evaluated the data from 10,499 patients aged <70 and 2,170 aged ≥70. All the efficacy endpoints (overall survival, disease-free survival, and time to treatment failure) were significantly improved for the experimental arm in the younger patients, but this benefit was lost in the older patients. A more recent and even larger ACCENT study was carried out to study the treatment outcomes in the very young patient with stage II and III colon cancer, those aged <40 and <50 (Sargent et al. 2010). This study involved 33,574 patients from 24 randomized controlled studies. Younger patients have significantly improved disease-free survival and overall survival rates compared to older patients. The investigators postulated that the improved survival was due to fewer competing causes of death.

The evidence of benefit in an elderly patient treated with an oxaliplatin-based adjuvant therapy is less consistent than that of adjuvant 5-fluorouracil. Results of subgroup analyses of two phase III trials were positive for benefit in one but negative for the other. Unfortunately, the population-based analyses also suggested that any benefit from adjuvant therapy was lost in the elderly age group.

15.4.3 Life Expectancy, Competing Mortality, and Cancer Recurrence

There are concerns that any survival benefits derived from adjuvant chemotherapy for the elderly patients may be truncated by a limited remaining life span or competing deaths. A fit 75-year-old person in the USA has an average life expectancy of 10–12 years (Arias 2010). The presence of coexisting illness after diagnosis of early colorectal cancer is associated with a reduction in life expectancy (Gross et al. 2006). Among men diagnosed with stage I colorectal cancer at 67 years of age, the life expectancy was 19.1 years if no coexisting illness, 12.4 years for 1–2 coexisting illnesses, and 7.6 years for 3 or more coexisting illnesses. A similar trend is reported for women. A large population-based analysis evaluated age and adjuvant chemotherapy use in 6,262 stage III colon cancer patients aged ≥65 (Schrag et al. 2001). About 33% of the patients had one comorbid condition and 13% had two or more. In spite of this, the investigators found that for patients aged ≥75, about 40% of patients were still alive at 5 years after surgery. Majority of the deaths that occurred are due to cancer. The investigators felt that these patients still have sufficient life expectancy to warrant consideration for adjuvant chemotherapy.

The rate of competing mortality from noncancer causes is probably around 10%. A large phase III study (INT 0089) comparing four different 5-fluorouracil-based adjuvant regimens for stage II and III colon cancer observed a 13% rate of noncancer deaths (Haller et al. 2005). A pooled analysis of seven randomized adjuvant trials for stage II and III colon cancer also reported that 13% of patients died without evidence of recurrence (Sargent et al. 2001a, b). A phase III study of elderly women with node-positive breast cancer randomized to adjuvant hormonal therapy versus observation observed that 9.1% of patients died without apparent relapses from cancer (Castiglione et al. 1990).

Patient data from 18 phase III adjuvant colon clinical studies were analyzed for the purpose of correlating 3-year disease-free survival to overall survival (Sargent et al. 2005). The investigators also recorded the recurrence rate of the cancer – 80% of the recurrences occurred in the first 3 years and nearly all by 5 years. This means that any recurrences that will occur would do so well within the remaining life expectancy of the elderly patient even when limited by comorbidities.

The life expectancy of a fit elderly cancer patient poses little contraindication for routine consideration for adjuvant chemotherapy. Even in the presence of coexisting illness, some elderly patients still have reasonable longevity to warrant a discussion regarding adjuvant chemotherapy. Moreover, majority of the cancer recurrences that occur do so within the first 3 years after diagnosis, and most of the patients that die do so from their cancer. Adjuvant chemotherapy may grant many well elderly patients a number of cancer-free years. These factors form compelling reasons to consider adjuvant chemotherapy for the majority of elderly patients.

15.5   Do Senior Cancer Patients Experience Greater Toxicity from Adjuvant Chemotherapy?

The senior patient poses a unique set of challenges to the cancer physician when contemplating potentially toxic chemotherapy for the patient. Age-associated factors such as presence of comorbid diseases, geriatric syndromes, impaired organ functions, diminished organ reserves, and altered pharmacokinetic and pharmacodynamics parameters may increase the risk of treatment-induced toxicity and impaired stress tolerance (Balducci and Extermann 2000; Lichtman 2003). As a result of these factors, physicians perceive that senior cancer patients are likely to suffer greater harm from treatment compared to younger patients. Unlike trying to extrapolate efficacy data in the metastatic to the curative setting, the author feels that it is reasonable to review the toxicity data in both the adjuvant and metastatic therapy. Perhaps one might even argue that toxicity data in the metastatic setting could have a higher "sensitivity" than those in the postoperative setting as these patients are not preselected for surgery, and they bear a greater burden of disease.

15.5.1 Toxicity Data of Fluoropyrimidine-Based Adjuvant Therapy

In the final report of the INT 0089 study, which compared four different adjuvant bolus 5-fluorouracil-based regimens, older patients had significantly higher rates of stomatitis and leucopenia (Haller et al. 2005). In spite of this, there was no difference in compliance between patients aged 40–70 and ≥70. Pooled data from seven randomized controlled adjuvant trials (five trials involving bolus 5-fluorouracil/leucovorin and two trials involving bolus 5-fluorouracil/levamisole) showed that age was not associated with the rate of grade 3 or higher nausea or emesis, stomatitis or diarrhea among treated patients (Sargent et al. 2001a, b). On the other hand, increased age (≥70 years) was significantly related to a higher rate of severe leucopenia in patients treated with 5-fluorouracil/levamisole (31% vs. 17%). Data from the SEER database suggested that hospitalization for complications (neutropenia, mucositis, diarrhea, bacteremia, sepsis, and dehydration) increased with increasing age: 7% in patients aged 65–79, 9% in 75–79, and 13% in 85–89 (Schrag et al. 2001).

In contrast, there are two studies that suggested the contrary. A 10-year report from a single US institution did not find any increase in toxicity among the older patients (Fata et al. 2002). Sixteen percent of the younger patients (<65 years) experienced grade 3–4 toxicity compared to 22% in the older patients ($p=0.420$). A safety analysis of the X-ACT study also failed to detect any difference in the safety profile of patients aged <65 or ≥65 when they were treated with the oral fluoropyrimidine – capecitabine (Scheithauer et al. 2003).

15.5.2 Toxicity Data of Fluoropyrimidine-Based Metastatic Therapy

Most of the studies involving 5-fluorouracil therapy for colorectal cancer patients in the metastatic setting reported some degree of greater toxicity encountered in the older patients. Commonly reported increased toxicity in the older patients included mucositis, leukopenia, and diarrhea (D'Andre et al. 2005; Blanke et al. 2011; Popescu et al. 1999; Stein et al. 1995; Zalcberg et al. 1998). Some studies even reported a higher rate of death in treated elderly patients. A multi-institutional phase III trial of 5-fluorouracil treatment for advanced colorectal cancer (Stein et al. 1995) found that patients 70 years or older were at significantly increased risk for severe toxicity compared to younger patients: any severe adverse event (58% vs. 36%), leukopenia (24% vs. 10%), diarrhea (24% vs. 14%), vomiting (15% vs. 5%), toxicity in more than 2 organ systems (10% vs. 3%), and treatment-related death (9% vs. 2%). Two hundred and forty-three patients with colorectal cancer were treated in a single Israeli center using the Mayo regimen, which comprised of bolus 5-fluorouracil/leucovorin×5 days and repeated once every 28 days (Tsalic et al. 2003). About equal number of patients were being treated with adjuvant and metastatic therapy. Major toxicities included neutropenic fever, mucositis, and diarrhea. Elderly patients (≥70) developed severe toxicities more frequently than younger patients: 24% versus 7%. Four out of 89 older patients (≥70 years) compared to 1 out of 154 younger patients died from treatment. A retrospective analysis of a large pool of patients from 22 European trials showed that infusional 5-fluorouracil in older patients (≥70 years) was not only superior in terms of efficacy but also safety when compared to bolus 5-fluorouracil (Folprecht et al. 2004). A trend to reduced 60-day mortality was observed in the elderly patients who received the infusion administration. A meta-analysis of more than 1,200 patients, which compared the efficacy and toxicity profiles of these two modalities of administration of 5-fluorouracil, reported similar findings of better efficacy and lesser toxicity with infusional 5-fluorouracil (Efficacy of intravenous continuous infusion of fluorouracil compared with bolus administration in advanced colorectal cancer. Meta-analysis Group In Cancer 1998).

Two large phase III studies have confirmed the equivalent efficacy, improved safety profile, and improved convenience of capecitabine compared with 5-fluorouracil/leucovorin in patients with metastatic colorectal cancer (Van Cutsem et al. 2004). A phase II Spanish study showed that capecitabine was effective and tolerable in patients aged 70 or older (Feliu et al. 2005). Other studies observed a lower tolerability with capecitabine in the frail elderly patients. When the Capecitabine Colorectal Cancer Group investigators evaluated the safety profile of capecitabine, they discovered that there was an increased incidence of grade 3 or worse adverse events, particularly those related to the gastrointestinal tract, among patients 80 years of age or older (Cassidy et al. 2002). The multivariate analysis suggested that it was not age per se but rather age-related impairment of renal function that was associated with increased toxicity. The recent MRC FOCUS2 study, which will be discussed in more details in the subsequent portion of this review, reported that capecitabine did not improve the quality of life compared with 5-fluorouracil in the frail elderly (Seymour et al. 2011).

15.5.3 Toxicity Data of Oxaliplatin-Based Adjuvant Therapy

A planned safety analysis in 1,864 patients with stage III colon patients who received adjuvant XELOX (CAPOX) or 5-fluorouracil/leucovorin therapy was recently reported (Schmoll et al. 2007). XELOX-treated patients experienced less frequent severe hematological but more frequent severe gastrointestinal toxicity when compared to the Mayo regimen (bolus 5-fluorouracil/leucovorin×5 days, repeated every 28 days). On the other hand, XELOX-treated patients developed more frequent severe hematological and less frequent severe gastrointestinal toxicity when compared to Roswell Park regimen (weekly 5-fluorouracil/leucovorin). Expectedly XELOX was associated with greater incidence of neurotoxicity and hand-foot syndrome when compared to either 5-fluorouracil/leucovorin regimens. The safety profiles of XELOX and 5-fluorouracil/leucovorin were analyzed in patients <65 and those ≥65 years in age. The highest rate of overall grade 3/4 toxicity, grade 3/4 diarrhea, and grade 3/4 dehydration and toxicity-related treatment discontinuation were seen in the older group of patients treated with XELOX.

In order to evaluate the tolerance of FOLFOX in elderly patients, safety data of 3,742 patients with colorectal cancer treated in the adjuvant, first-line, and second-line settings were reviewed (Goldberg et al. 2006). Of these patients, more than half were treated for adjuvant reasons, a quarter in the first-line setting and the remaining quarter in second-line setting. Older patients (≥70 years) experienced higher rates of grade 3 or worse neutropenia and thrombocytopenia. It is reassuring to know that the increased incidence of severe hematological toxicity did not translate into any increase in the overall incidence of grade ≥3 toxicity, infection, or mortality. Additionally, dose intensity did not differ by age. Another earlier analysis also examined the safety data of colorectal cancer patients treated in the same three settings: adjuvant, first-line, and second-line (Tabah-Fisch et al. 2002). However, in this instance, the great majority (78%) of patients were treated in the adjuvant setting. There was an increase in some toxicity (stomatitis, neutropenia, and thrombocytopenia) but only in the older patients who were pretreated. The overall incidence of severe toxicities was similar; increasing age did not affect the efficacy/safety ratio. A special concern regarding oxaliplatin treatment is the neurotoxicity. In both of the studies cited here, older age was not associated with any increased rate of severe neurological events.

Two population-based studies did not observe any increase in adverse events between ages. In fact, one of the studies observed that treated elderly patients had fewer adverse events than younger patients (Kahn et al. 2010). The CanCORS study found that among patients treated with adjuvant chemotherapy, the adjusted rate of late adverse events was lowest in the oldest patients (≥75 years). The investigators believe that the fewer adverse events were due to fewer older patients being treated with more toxic regimens and fewer older patients being able to complete their chemotherapy. The ACCENT study tried to evaluate the effects of adjuvant therapy in the young colorectal cancer patients (Sargent et al. 2010). Although the young patients had improved disease-free and overall survival compared to the older patients, there were no clinically meaningful differences in adverse events between the ages.

15.5.4 Toxicity Data of Oxaliplatin-Based Metastatic Therapy

Interestingly, a series of phase II studies of oral fluoropyrimidines plus oxaliplatin as first-line treatment for elderly colorectal cancer patients (≥70 years) did not show any increase in treatment toxicity (Comella et al. 2005; Feliu et al. 2006; Rosati et al. 2005). However, in two of three studies cited, there was manipulation of capecitabine dose – one study adopted graduated dosing and the other employed dose adjustment according to creatinine clearance. In another phase II study, a post hoc analysis of the efficacy and safety of CAPOX in patients <65 years of age versus patient ≥65 years of age observed that there were no differences in either efficacy, toxicity, dose reductions, or treatment withdrawals between the 2 age categories (Twelves et al. 2005b).

The underrepresentation of older people in clinical trials has persistently prevented investigators from interpreting the data accurately. This problem appears to have been circumvented for the first time in the largest ever randomized controlled trial to have selectively enrolled frail older adults with advanced colorectal cancer (Seymour et al. 2011). The FOCUS2 (Fluorouracil, Oxaliplatin, CPT11[irinotecan]: Use and Sequencing) study recruited 459 elderly patients (median age was 74 years) with 43% of patients older than 75 years and 13% older than 80. Less than a quarter of the patients had performance status of 0, half had a performance status of 1, and more than a quarter a performance status of 2. The study had a 2×2 factorial design, and patients were randomized into one of the four treatment arms: 5-fluorouracil, FOLFOX, capecitabine, or CAPOX. This trial included innovative designs to address the gaps encountered in earlier elderly cancer patient studies – starting doses were reduced to 80% of standard doses, comprehensive geriatric health assessments were performed, and outcome measurements incorporated subjective and objective measures of benefit and harm. The investigators found that the addition of oxaliplatin improved the progression-free survival in a nonsignificant way but did not significantly increase any grade 3 or worse toxicity.

On the other hand, subset analysis of a large phase III study comparing FOLFOX with 5-fluorouracil/leucovorin in 420 patients with metastatic colorectal cancer reported an increased rate of grade 3 or worse diarrhea among older patients (>65 years) when compared to their younger counterparts (de Gramont et al. 2000).

15.5.5 Summary

Increased severe toxicity in the older patients from fluoropyrimidine therapy is reported more often in the metastatic setting. They most commonly include stomatitis, neutropenia, and diarrhea. In spite of this, the elderly patients generally appear to be as likely to tolerate the treatment as their younger counterparts. Infrequently an increased rate of treatment-related deaths has been reported. These toxicities are probably related to bolus 5-fluorouracil, which makes protracted infusion the preferred mode of administration in the elderly patient.

Capecitabine is highly tolerable in many aspects when compared to bolus 5-fluorouracil. It is also more convenient being an orally administered drug. However, use of capecitabine in the elderly may be associated with greater toxicity in the frail senior or those with impaired renal function.

Toxicity appears to be more frequently reported for XELOX compared to FOLFOX. One large phase III study observed that XELOX was associated with increased severe toxicity and treatment withdrawal in the older patients. In contrast, FOLFOX did not appear to cause any major unfavorable efficacy/safety ratio in the elderly patients. This suggests that the use of capecitabine whether alone or in combination with oxaliplatin should be carefully considered in the elderly. There appears to be a greater increase in severe hematological and gastrointestinal adverse events compared to neurological toxicity in elderly patients who received oxaliplatin-based treatments.

15.6   How Should Senior Patients with Resected Stage II Colon Be Managed?

The QUASAR trial was the single largest randomized control trial that enrolled patients with stage II colorectal cancer to evaluate the benefit of adjuvant chemotherapy (Gray et al. 2007). The investigators estimated that the absolute benefit with

5-fluorouracil-based chemotherapy for this group of low risk patients is 3.6%. Although the pooled analysis of four NSABP adjuvant trials also demonstrated an improved outcome with adjuvant chemotherapy, this analysis was criticized for its heterogeneity in treatment and unconventional statistical method (Mamounas et al. 1999). Apart from these two positive studies, several other phase III, pooled analyses and population-based studies addressing the same question were unable to find any benefit of adjuvant chemotherapy in stage II cancer patients (Gill et al. 2004; IMPACT B2 1999; Moertel et al. 1995; O'Connor et al. 2011; Schrag et al. 2002). Of note is a very large but recent population-based study involving data of 24,847 patients with stage II colon cancer who underwent colectomy from 1992 to 2005 (O'Connor et al. 2011). Majority (68%) of the patients were over the age of 75 years at diagnosis. Majority (75%) of patients had one or more poor prognostic features. Twenty percent of the patients received adjuvant chemotherapy. The analysis failed to find any improvement in survival regardless of the presence or absence of poor prognostic features.

In the first report of the MOSAIC study, the addition of oxaliplatin to infusional 5-fluoruracil significantly improved the 3-year disease-free survival of stage II and III colon cancer: 78.2% versus 72.9% (Andre et al. 2004). A test of interaction showed no significant interaction between stage and treatment leading the investigators to suggest that adjuvant treatment benefitted both stage II and III colon cancer. However, in the updated 6-year report, the survival curves of the patients with stage II disease in the experimental and control arms overlapped exactly (Andre et al. 2009). In a similarly designed study, the NSABP C07 investigators used oxaliplatin plus bolus instead of infusional 5-fluorouracil for the experimental arm of treatment (Kuebler et al. 2007). Likewise, they found that the oxaliplatin/5-fluorouracil combination significantly improved disease-free survival and no interaction between treatment effect and stage. However, the investigators acknowledged that the study was not powered to evaluate efficacy in patient subsets so no conclusions could be drawn.

The current NCCN guidelines (NCCN Guidelines 2011) recommend that high-risk stage II disease (e.g., high-grade tumor, T4, lymphovascular invasion, perineural infiltration, bowel obstruction, perforated or less than 12 lymph nodes sampled) should be considered for adjuvant chemotherapy as for stage III cancer. For low-risk stage II disease, appropriate options would include observation, clinical trial, or single-agent fluoropyrimidine treatment.

It can be seen that despite the NCC guidelines, the role of adjuvant therapy after surgery for stage II colon cancer remains questionable and the choice of optimal regimen remains controversial. The evidence regarding the use of 5-fluorouracil adjuvant therapy in stage II colon remains conflicting, and the magnitude of benefit, if present, is estimated to be at best 5%. The current recommended use of oxaliplatin-based adjuvant therapy in high-risk stage II disease is primarily based on extrapolated benefit from stage III disease rather than on good phase III evidence. This lack of consistent and reliable data regarding adjuvant chemotherapy in stage II disease makes it even more difficult to know if such a treatment is truly meaningful in the elderly subgroup.

15.7   What Are the Implications of Lower Treatment Doses and Shorter Duration?

In an earlier section of this chapter, which discussed the pattern of use of adjuvant chemotherapy in the elderly cancer patients, it was noted that older patients were often prescribed a less toxic regimen, they often received dose reductions, and they frequently do not complete the planned duration of treatment. Does this compromise the efficacy of treatment? Due to the paucity of data in this area, the author will review studies in both adjuvant and metastatic settings and in both colon and noncolon cancers.

The Capecitabine Colorectal Cancer Study Group investigators evaluated the impact of dose modification of capecitabine or 5-fluorouracil in 1,207 patients with advanced colorectal cancer (Cassidy et al. 2002). They found a statistically nonsignificant 30% increase in risk of disease progression or death in patients receiving 5-fluorouracil/leucovorin who required a dose reduction of 49–64% of baseline. On the other hand, dose reduction of capecitabine to either 75% or 50% of baseline due to adverse events did not compromise efficacy. A small phase II study also found that higher 5-fluorouracil dose intensity was associated with a clinical response (Grem et al. 1993). An analysis based on the SEER database evaluated the effect of premature discontinuation of adjuvant therapy in elderly (≥65 years) stage III cancer on survival (Neugut et al. 2006). The investigators discovered that more than 30% of elderly patients stopped treatment early (1–4 months). The risk of death (overall and cancer specific) in the group that received a shorter duration of treatment was nearly twice higher than those who completed 5–7 months of treatment.

A retrospective analysis of the role of dose level of CMF (cyclophosphamide/methotrexate/5-fluorouracil) in postoperative adjuvant and in palliative chemotherapy for breast cancer showed a clear dose-response relationship (Bonadonna and Valagussa 1981). Chemotherapy was only useful when delivered at ≥85% of the planned dose.

Studies involving small cell lung cancer demonstrated that higher doses of chemotherapy were associated with higher response and survival rates (Arriagada et al. 1993; Findlay et al. 1991).

Dose reduction appears to compromise the efficacy of 5-fluorouracil but not capecitabine. This could be due to the preferential activation of capecitabine in tumor through thymidine phosphorylase. This mechanism may generate up to 20 times the concentration of 5-fluorouracil within the tumor cells compared to the plasma compartment (Schuller et al. 2000). A shortened duration of adjuvant therapy appears to be associated with a higher risk of death.

15.8   Which Senior Cancer Patients Should Be Prescribed Adjuvant Chemotherapy and What Regimen Should Be Used?

It is recognized that the elderly population is a very heterogeneous population with varying degrees of coexisting diseases and age-related conditions, physical fitness and performance, mental and emotional state, organ reserve and impairment, and social and economic support. The survey by Keating et al. demonstrates that physicians are comfortable in making decisions for elderly patients at the two ends of the spectrum – they are unanimous and willing to recommend chemotherapy for the fit 80-year-old and are just as unanimous and willing to forego chemotherapy for 80-year-old with severe comorbidity (Keating et al. 2008). Physicians tend to differ widely on recommendations for patients who are in between the two extreme groups. Are there tools to help physicians select the right patients and can these tools be used in the elderly cancer population?

Physicians caring for senior patients have developed a multidimensional geriatric screening tool – the Comprehensive Geriatric Assessment (CGA) aimed to improve the process, outcome, and cost-effectiveness of care for this special patient population (Wieland and Hirth 2003). The basic components of the CGA are a medical assessment, an assessment of functioning, psychological assessment, social assessment, and environmental assessment. There is extensive and robust evidence supporting the use of the CGA in the care of elderly patients in both the hospital and community settings (Ferrucci et al. 2003). Hurria and colleagues conducted prechemotherapy CGAs in elderly cancer patients from seven institutions to determine if such a screening could predict severe toxicity. They found that the functional and social variables in the CGA in addition to tumor type, treatment regimens, and initial doses were predictive of severe toxicity (Hurria et al. 2010). A recent review article on the recent studies evaluating the utility of CGA in older cancer patients demonstrates that the CGA is able to predict morbidity and mortality, and discover problems relevant to cancer care in this population of patient (Extermann and Hurria 2007). A retrospective analysis of CGA data collected from 249 cancer patients aged ≥70 treated at the National Cancer Center Singapore was performed (Kanesvaran et al. 2011). Based on results from their multivariate analysis, the investigators developed a simple nomogram to predict overall survival. They found that their model was able to predict overall survival over 3 years with relatively good accuracy. To the investigators' knowledge, this is the first study to evaluate the use of CGA prospectively in an Asian context.

Three stages of aging can be recognized: (1) group 1 patients are fit (functionally independent and without any comorbidity), (2) group 2 patients are in-between (≥1 impaired function in the Instrumental Activities of Daily Living, 1–2 comorbid conditions), and (3) group 3 patients are frail (≥1 impaired function in the Activities of Daily Living, ≥3 comorbid conditions, ≥1 geriatric syndrome) (Balducci and Extermann 2000). Group 1 patients are potential candidates for full-dose life-prolonging anticancer treatment, and group 3 patients may only benefit from supportive management. Group 2 patients whose average life expectancy exceeds the life expectancy from cancer could be considered for tailored-dose strategy or less toxic regimen. Group 2 patients whose average life expectancy is less than life expectancy from cancer should be considered for best supportive care. Indeed, the FOCUS2 study adopted an attenuated dose strategy in a group of frail elderly patients (Seymour et al. 2011). The rapid recruitment of patients ahead of target in this study testifies to the readiness of physicians and their patients to accept treatment and the feasibility of such a treatment even in the compromised elderly cancer patients.

Applying the management algorithm described by Balducci and Extermann to the postoperative management of stage III colon cancer in the older patients would translate into the following recommendations: Group 1 patients could be offered adjuvant FOLFOX or CAPOX, group 2 patients could be considered for infusional 5-fluorouracil or capecitabine, and group 3 patients could be observed. However, physicians should remain cognizant of the scarcity of data on the use of FOLFOX in patients over 75 when prescribing it to the elderly patients. Elderly patients receiving capecitabine should have their renal function carefully monitored and the capecitabine dose adjusted according to the creatinine clearance (Cassidy et al. 2002; Poole et al. 2002). Investigators from Korea were able to demonstrate the feasibility of using a tailored-dose approach in prescribing adjuvant capecitabine in patients 70 years or older in age (Chang et al. 2011). The patients started with an initial dose at 80% of standard dose. Dose modification for the subsequent cycles of treatment was adjusted according to the severity of toxicity experienced during the first cycle. This strategy allowed half of the 82 patients enrolled to successfully complete the whole treatment while achieving ≥80% relative dose intensity.

Conclusion

The population is aging and colorectal cancer is associated with aging. Although there are established clinical practice guidelines for adjuvant therapy of resected stage III colon cancer, the elderly cancer patients tend to be undertreated due to concerns regarding fitness, coexisting conditions, and longevity. The data suggests that fit older patients have a long life expectancy and can derive the same magnitude of benefit as younger patients. Likewise, fit elderly patients appear to tolerate the toxicity of treatment in spite of some reports of increased rates of leucopenia, stomatitis, and diarrhea. Hence, it is warranted for physicians to recommend the standard treatment for the fit elderly colon cancer patient.

Clinical trial data regarding the efficacy/safety ratio of treatment in the frail elderly are lacking. In the absence of sufficient data, the routine use of a geriatric assessment could provide many advantages: (1) predicting life expectancy, (2) predicting risk of severe adverse events, (3) recognizing reversible conditions, (4) assessing functional reserves, and (5) developing a standardized management approach.

More research and a better definition are needed in the area of elderly people with "in-between" fitness. Better trial designs are necessary in order to carry out such research successfully. The FOCUS2 trial lends hope that more elderly-specific studies will emerge in the near future. Perhaps the usual clinical outcomes in adjuvant studies also need to be redefined for this group of patients – quality of life and relapse-free survival may be more sufficiently meaningful sufficient endpoints compared to the "gold standard" overall survival.

As the cancer physicians begin to care for more and more elderly cancer patients, there is a need to meld together geriatric and oncologic principles, adopt a multidisciplinary approach, and individualize the therapy.

15.9   A Commentary on Adjuvant Chemotherapy
         in Colorectal Cancer for Elderly Patients

Donald Poon

A cursory Pubmed online search yielded 85 published papers with titles or abstract text containing the term "elderly cancer patients" in the 50-year period 1951–2001. This is a relatively parsimonious harvest compared to the 225 publications in the last 10 years from 2001 to present (Pubmed online search 2011). Clinicians' interest has evidently increased with empirical improvement in output of academic publications on care of elderly cancer patients; this is also apparent in Singapore with the formation of clinical programs and common interest groups in the field of geriatric oncology. This interest is fuelled by a rising trend of total cancer incidence across all age groups and a rapidly ageing population in most developed countries especially Singapore with 9.3% of the population above 65 years old currently. In 2030, the latter proportion is expected to reach 25% in Singapore. Coupled with the fact that the age-specific incidence of colorectal cancer rises sharply after age 50 (Singapore Cancer Registry 2005–2009; Singapore Department of Statistics 2011), these 2 factors form a potent recipe for a formidable clinical conundrum – the application of adjuvant chemotherapy in up to 3,000 elderly patients with stage 2 or 3 colorectal cancer per year by 2030 in Singapore. Reiterating the imperative need to produce practical solutions to this conundrum is a rhetorical understatement.

Is there at present a cogent platform conducive for a comprehensive solution to this conundrum? As Dr. Ong, the author of the chapter on adjuvant chemotherapy in this monograph, rightly concluded, the crux of the matter is identifying who among the elderly patients will benefit from chemotherapy after surgery for colorectal cancers. While we are doing well in prognostication and prediction of treatment outcome based on tumor-related factors such as TNM staging and K-ras mutation status, we have floundered in patient-related factors. Three compounding factors in the form of (1) prevailing political correctness overpowering rational reasoning, (2) publication bias in the presentation of available medical evidence, and (3) the compartmentalization of the practice of medicine have all colluded to prevent us clinicians from developing a coherent approach to appropriate patient selection.

A juror is disallowed from reading all newspaper coverage of the trial he is involved in, for fear of being unduly influenced by popular opinion that may confer a bias resulting in hasty prejudging and unfair assessment of the evidence presented in court. However, the situation in discussion here cannot be more different. The fear of being labeled an "ageist" is equivalent to being labeled with similitudes such as "racist." This climate of being politically correct is pervasive and has influenced broad-based opinion in the optimal management of the elderly cancer patient (an unforgivable term in some circles; the better accepted form being "senior adult oncology patient"). Take, for example, the interpretation of the following piece of information. The changes in cancer incidence and mortality have been worse in the elderly than in younger patients based on North American SEER database. From 1950 to 1990, the incidence of cancer (all sites and types combined) increased by 26% in patients older than 65 but by only 10% in younger patients. The overall cancer mortality in that period increased by

15% in older patients and decreased by 5% in younger patients (Lyman 1998). It will be politically correct to conclude that we are neglecting the senior adults in oncology. But as pointed out earlier, attention to elderly cancer patients has increased over the decades, and this is anecdotally so in actual clinical practice. Even women aged 80 or more are being referred for adjuvant chemotherapy after surgery for colorectal cancers. Could not it be that the increased mortality is a result of a rising trend of elderly patients receiving cytotoxics with attendant increase in complications possibly curtailing survival? This is certainly a plausible postulation, but when openly expressed, it may draw much criticism in these times.

As popularized by Mark Twain and attributed to Disraeli, there are three kinds of lies – lies, damned lies, and statistics. The wrong perception that all elderly colorectal patients should be offered adjuvant chemotherapy is bolstered by selective positioning of positive clinical trials and meta-analyses in the medical literature (Sargent et al. 2001a, b; Muss et al. 2007). This has been adroitly addressed by local clinicians (Tan et al. 2010; Koh and Seow-Choen 2006.) who advised that the practice advocated in the prevailing published evidence is based on tenuous grounds mainly because the elderly patient populations were inappropriately and inadequately represented in the individual studies that were used for the above meta-analyses. Publication bias is rife. Data from two separate European phase II trials conducted by EORTC (European Organisation for Research and Treatment of Cancer) and the Italian NHLCSG studying the tolerability of non-anthracycline-based chemotherapy regimens which were supposedly relatively innocuous in frail elderly patients with lymphoma was never published. Both studies were discontinued early due to excessive toxic deaths (>25%) after accrual of less than 30 patients (Extermann 2006).

The complex interaction of comorbidities, tumor biology and molecular profile, physiological changes in ageing, and genetic factors imposes an interface that demands a multidisciplinary approach. With subspecialization in medical practice, coordinating such an approach is formidable and expensive but nevertheless necessary to identify those suitable for adjuvant chemotherapy. It is a work in progress. The comprehensive geriatric assessment (CGA) has been adopted by the CALGB (Cancer Leukemia Group B) for baseline assessment of all elderly patients enrolled in their clinical trials. This is a major step forward in accurate clinical profiling of these elderly patients in order for clinicians to better decide if the trial results are applicable to specific elderly patients with cancer under their care in clinical practice.

In conclusion, no one can proclaim with alacrity that all elderly colorectal patients should be offered adjuvant chemotherapy with undoubted benefit based on current available information. It is wrong to distort facts to fit an agenda. It seems that current opinion starts by begging the question thereby committing the fallacy of *petitio principii*. I know of only one person who can define as he wishes (Carroll 1872).

> "But 'glory' doesn't mean 'a nice knock-down argument'," Alice objected.
>
> "When I use a word," Humpty Dumpty said, in rather a scornful tone, "it means just what I choose it to mean—neither more nor less."
>
> "The question is," said Alice, "whether you can make words mean so many different things."
>
> "The question is," said Humpty Dumpty, "which is to be master – that's all."

Donald Poon, Raffles Cancer Centre, Founding President, Society of Geriatric, Oncology, Singapore

References

Abrams TA, Brightly R, Mao J et al (2011) Patterns of adjuvant chemotherapy use in a population-based cohort of patients with resected stage II or III colon cancer. J Clin Oncol 29:3255–3262

Allegra CJ, Yothers G, O'Connell MJ et al (2011) Phase III trial assessing bevacizumab in stages II and III carcinoma of the colon: results of NSABP protocol C-08. J Clin Oncol 29:11–16

Ananda S, Field KM, Kosmider S et al (2008) Patient age and comorbidity are major determinants of adjuvant chemotherapy use for stage III colon cancer in routine clinical practice. J Clin Oncol 26:4516–4517; author reply 4517–4518

Andre T, Boni C, Mounedji-Boudiaf L et al (2004) Oxaliplatin, fluorouracil, and leucovorin as adjuvant treatment for colon cancer. N Engl J Med 350:2343–2351

Andre T, Boni C, Navarro M et al (2009) Improved overall survival with oxaliplatin, fluorouracil, and leucovorin as adjuvant treatment in stage II or III colon cancer in the MOSAIC trial. J Clin Oncol 27:3109–3116

Aparicio T, Desrame J, Lecomte T et al (2003) Oxaliplatin- or irinotecan-based chemotherapy for metastatic colorectal cancer in the elderly. Br J Cancer 89:1439–1444

Arias E (2010) United States life tables, 2006. National Vital Statistics Reports, Vol 58, No 21

Arriagada R, Le Chevalier T, Pignon JP et al (1993) Initial chemotherapeutic doses and survival in patients with limited small-cell lung cancer. N Engl J Med 329:1848–1852

Balducci L, Extermann M (2000) Management of cancer in the older person: a practical approach. Oncologist 5:224–237

Blanke CD, Bot BM, Thomas DM et al (2011) Impact of young age on treatment efficacy and safety in advanced colorectal cancer: a pooled analysis of patients from nine first-line phase III chemotherapy trials. J Clin Oncol 29:2781–2786

Bonadonna G, Valagussa P (1981) Dose-response effect of adjuvant chemotherapy in breast cancer. N Engl J Med 304:10–15

Carroll L (1872) Through the looking-glass. Hayes Barton Press, Raleigh, p 72. ISBN ISBN 1593772165

Cassidy J, Twelves C, Van Cutsem E et al (2002) First-line oral capecitabine therapy in metastatic colorectal cancer: a favorable safety profile compared with intravenous 5-fluorouracil/leucovorin. Ann Oncol 13:566–575

Castiglione M, Gelber RD, Goldhirsch A (1990) Adjuvant systemic therapy for breast cancer in the elderly: competing causes of mortality. International Breast Cancer Study Group. J Clin Oncol 8:519–526

Chang HJ, Lee KW, Kim JH et al (2011) Adjuvant capecitabine chemotherapy using a tailored-dose strategy in elderly patients with colon cancer. Ann Oncol. doi:10.1093/annonc/mdr329

Choo PW, Lee KS, Owen RE et al (1990) Singapore – an ageing society. Singapore Med J 31:486–488

Choo PW, Sahadevan S, Chee YC et al (1991) Health care services for the elderly – a Singapore perspective. Singapore Med J 32:319–323

Comella P, Natale D, Farris A et al (2005) Capecitabine plus oxaliplatin for the first-line treatment of elderly patients with metastatic colorectal carcinoma: final results of the Southern Italy Cooperative Oncology Group Trial 0108. Cancer 104:282–289

D'Andre S, Sargent DJ, Cha SS et al (2005) 5-Fluorouracil-based chemotherapy for advanced colorectal cancer in elderly patients: a north central cancer treatment group study. Clin Colorectal Cancer 4:325–331

de Gramont A, Figer A, Seymour M et al (2000) Leucovorin and fluorouracil with or without oxaliplatin as first-line treatment in advanced colorectal cancer. J Clin Oncol 18:2938–2947

Dobie SA, Baldwin LM, Dominitz JA et al (2006) Completion of therapy by Medicare patients with stage III colon cancer. J Natl Cancer Inst 98:610–619

Efficacy of adjuvant fluorouracil and folinic acid in B2 colon cancer. International Multicentre Pooled Analysis of B2 Colon Cancer Trials (IMPACT B2) Investigators (1999) J Clin Oncol 17:1356–1363

Efficacy of adjuvant fluorouracil and folinic acid in colon cancer. International Multicentre Pooled Analysis of Colon Cancer Trials (IMPACT) investigators (1995) Lancet 345:939–944

Efficacy of intravenous continuous infusion of fluorouracil compared with bolus administration in advanced colorectal cancer. Meta-analysis Group In Cancer (1998) J Clin Oncol 16: 301–308

Extermann M (2006) Comorbidity and cancer. American Society of Clinical Oncology (ASCO) Educational book

Extermann M, Hurria A (2007) Comprehensive geriatric assessment for older patients with cancer. J Clin Oncol 25:1824–1831

Fata F, Mirza A, Craig G et al (2002) Efficacy and toxicity of adjuvant chemotherapy in elderly patients with colon carcinoma: a 10-year experience of the Geisinger Medical Center. Cancer 94:1931–1938

Feliu J, Escudero P, Llosa F et al (2005) Capecitabine as first-line treatment for patients older than 70 years with metastatic colorectal cancer: an oncopaz cooperative group study. J Clin Oncol 23:3104–3111

Feliu J, Salud A, Escudero P et al (2006) XELOX (capecitabine plus oxaliplatin) as first-line treatment for elderly patients over 70 years of age with advanced colorectal cancer. Br J Cancer 94:969–975

Ferrucci L, Guralnik JM, Cavazzini C et al (2003) The frailty syndrome: a critical issue in geriatric oncology. Crit Rev Oncol Hematol 46:127–137

Findlay MP, Griffin AM, Raghavan D et al (1991) Retrospective review of chemotherapy for small cell lung cancer in the elderly: does the end justify the means? Eur J Cancer 27:1597–1601

Folprecht G, Cunningham D, Ross P et al (2004) Efficacy of 5-fluorouracil-based chemotherapy in elderly patients with metastatic colorectal cancer: a pooled analysis of clinical trials. Ann Oncol 15:1330–1338

Fried TR, Bradley EH, Towle VR et al (2002) Understanding the treatment preferences of seriously ill patients. N Engl J Med 346:1061–1066

Gill S, Loprinzi CL, Sargent DJ et al (2004) Pooled analysis of fluorouracil-based adjuvant therapy for stage II and III colon cancer: who benefits and by how much? J Clin Oncol 22:1797–1806

Goldberg RM, Tabah-Fisch I, Bleiberg H et al (2006) Pooled analysis of safety and efficacy of oxaliplatin plus fluorouracil/leucovorin administered bimonthly in elderly patients with colorectal cancer. J Clin Oncol 24:4085–4091

Gray R, Barnwell J, McConkey C et al (2007) Adjuvant chemotherapy versus observation in patients with colorectal cancer: a randomised study. Lancet 370:2020–2029

Grem JL, Jordan E, Robson ME et al (1993) Phase II study of fluorouracil, leucovorin, and interferon alfa-2a in metastatic colorectal carcinoma. J Clin Oncol 11:1737–1745

Gross CP, McAvay GJ, Krumholz HM et al (2006) The effect of age and chronic illness on life expectancy after a diagnosis of colorectal cancer: implications for screening. Ann Intern Med 145:646–653

NCCN Clinical Practice Guidelines in Oncology [NCCN Guidelines] (2011) Colon cancer version 1.2012. http://www.nccn.org/professionals/physician_gls/f_guidelines.asp. Accessed 2 Nov 2011

Haller DG, Catalano PJ, Macdonald JS et al (2005) Phase III study of fluorouracil, leucovorin, and levamisole in high-risk stage II and III colon cancer: final report of Intergroup 0089. J Clin Oncol 23:8671–8678

Haller DG, Cassidy J, Tabernero J et al (2010) Efficacy findings from a randomized phase III trial of capecitabine plus oxaliplatin versus bolus 5-FU/LV for stage III colon cancer (NO16968): no impact of age on disease-free survival (DFS). J Clin Oncol 28(15s): abstract 3521

Hamel MB, Teno JM, Goldman L et al (1999) Patient age and decisions to withhold life-sustaining treatments from seriously ill, hospitalized adults. SUPPORT Investigators. Study to Understand Prognoses and Preferences for Outcomes and Risks of Treatment. Ann Intern Med 130:116–125

Hurria A, Togawa K, Mohile SG et al (2010) Predicting chemotherapy toxicity in older adults with cancer: a prospective 500 patient multicenter study. J Clin Oncol 28(15s): abstract 9001

Hutchins LF, Unger JM, Crowley JJ et al (1999) Underrepresentation of patients 65 years of age or older in cancer-treatment trials. N Engl J Med 341:2061–2067

Iwashyna TJ, Lamont EB (2002) Effectiveness of adjuvant fluorouracil in clinical practice: a population-based cohort study of elderly patients with stage III colon cancer. J Clin Oncol 20:3992–3998

Jackson McCleary NA, Meyerhardt J, Green E et al (2009) Impact of older age on the efficacy of newer adjuvant therapies in >12,500 patients (pts) with stage II/III colon cancer: findings from the ACCENT Database. J Clin Oncol 27(15s): abstract 4010

Jessup JM, Stewart A, Greene FL et al (2005) Adjuvant chemotherapy for stage III colon cancer: implications of race/ethnicity, age, and differentiation. JAMA 294:2703–2711

Kahn KL, Adams JL, Weeks JC et al (2010) Adjuvant chemotherapy use and adverse events among older patients with stage III colon cancer. JAMA 303:1037–1045

Kanesvaran R, Li H, Koo KN et al (2011) Analysis of prognostic factors of comprehensive geriatric assessment and development of a clinical scoring system in elderly Asian patients with cancer. J Clin Oncol 29:3620–3627

Keating NL, Landrum MB, Klabunde CN et al (2008) Adjuvant chemotherapy for stage III colon cancer: do physicians agree about the importance of patient age and comorbidity? J Clin Oncol 26:2532–2537

Koh PK, Seow-Choen F (2006) Multicentre prospective randomized trials are not always relevant to surgeons. ANZ J Surg 76:286–287

Kuebler JP, Wieand HS, O'Connell MJ et al (2007) Oxaliplatin combined with weekly bolus fluorouracil and leucovorin as surgical adjuvant chemotherapy for stage II and III colon cancer: results from NSABP C-07. J Clin Oncol 25:2198–2204

Lembersky BC, Wieand HS, Petrelli NJ et al (2006) Oral uracil and tegafur plus leucovorin compared with intravenous fluorouracil and leucovorin in stage II and III carcinoma of the colon: results from National Surgical Adjuvant Breast and Bowel Project Protocol C-06. J Clin Oncol 24:2059–2064

Lichtman SM (2003) Guidelines for the treatment of elderly cancer patients. Cancer Control 10:445–453

Lyman GH (1998) Cancer care in the elderly. Cancer Control 5:347–354

Mamounas E, Wieand S, Wolmark N et al (1999) Comparative efficacy of adjuvant chemotherapy in patients with Dukes' B versus Dukes' C colon cancer: results from four National Surgical Adjuvant Breast and Bowel Project adjuvant studies (C-01, C-02, C-03, and C-04). J Clin Oncol 17:1349–1355

Meropol NJ, Egleston BL, Buzaglo JS et al (2008) Cancer patient preferences for quality and length of life. Cancer 113:3459–3466

Moertel CG, Fleming TR, Macdonald JS et al (1990) Levamisole and fluorouracil for adjuvant therapy of resected colon carcinoma. N Engl J Med 322:352–358

Moertel CG, Fleming TR, Macdonald JS et al (1995) Intergroup study of fluorouracil plus levamisole as adjuvant therapy for stage II/Dukes' B2 colon cancer. J Clin Oncol 13:2936–2943

Muss HB, Biganzoli L, Sargent DJ, Aapro M (2007) Adjuvant therapy in the elderly: making the right decision. J Clin Oncol 25(14):1870–1875

Neugut AI, Matasar M, Wang X et al (2006) Duration of adjuvant chemotherapy for colon cancer and survival among the elderly. J Clin Oncol 24:2368–2375

Newcomb PA, Carbone PP (1993) Cancer treatment and age: patient perspectives. J Natl Cancer Inst 85:1580–1584

NIH Consensus Conference (1990) Adjuvant therapy for patients with colon and rectal cancer. JAMA 264:1444–1450

O'Connor ES, Greenblatt DY, LoConte NK et al (2011) Adjuvant chemotherapy for stage II colon cancer with poor prognostic features. J Clin Oncol 29:3381–3388

Poole C, Gardiner J, Twelves C et al (2002) Effect of renal impairment on the pharmacokinetics and tolerability of capecitabine (Xeloda) in cancer patients. Cancer Chemother Pharmacol 49:225–234

Popescu RA, Norman A, Ross PJ et al (1999) Adjuvant or palliative chemotherapy for colorectal cancer in patients 70 years or older. J Clin Oncol 17:2412–2418

Pubmed online search for publications whose title or abstract text contain the terms "elderly cancer patients" [Internet] (2011) [Updated 2011 Dec 5; cited 2011 Dec 5]. Available from: http://www.ncbi.nlm.nih.gov/pubmed/

Quipourt V, Jooste V, Cottet V et al (2011) Comorbidities alone do not explain the undertreatment of colorectal cancer in older adults: a French population-based study. J Am Geriatr Soc 59:694–698

Rosati G, Cordio S, Tucci A et al (2005) Phase II trial of oxaliplatin and tegafur/uracil and oral folinic acid for advanced or metastatic colorectal cancer in elderly patients. Oncology 69:122–129

Saltz LB, Niedzwiecki D, Hollis D et al (2007) Irinotecan fluorouracil plus leucovorin is not superior to fluorouracil plus leucovorin alone as adjuvant treatment for stage III colon cancer: results of CALGB 89803. J Clin Oncol 25:3456–3461

Sargent DJ, Goldberg RM, Jacobson SD et al (2001) A pooled analysis of adjuvant chemotherapy for resected colon cancer in elderly patients. N Engl J Med 345:1091–1097

Sargent DJ, Wieand HS, Haller DG et al (2005) Disease-free survival versus overall survival as a primary end point for adjuvant colon cancer studies: individual patient data from 20,898 patients on 18 randomized trials. J Clin Oncol 23:8664–8670

Sargent DJ, Yothers GA, Green E et al (2010) Benefits and adverse events (AEs) in younger (Y) (age <50) versus older patients (pts) receiving adjuvant chemotherapy (AT) for colon cancer (CC): findings from the 33,574 pt ACCENT dataset. J Clin Olcol 28(15s): abstract 3523

Scheithauer W, McKendrick J, Begbie S et al (2003) Oral capecitabine as an alternative to i.v. 5-fluorouracil-based adjuvant therapy for colon cancer: safety results of a randomized, phase III trial. Ann Oncol 14:1735–1743

Schmoll HJ, Cartwright T, Tabernero J et al (2007) Phase III trial of capecitabine plus oxaliplatin as adjuvant therapy for stage III colon cancer: a planned safety analysis in 1,864 patients. J Clin Oncol 25:102–109

Schrag D, Cramer LD, Bach PB et al (2001) Age and adjuvant chemotherapy use after surgery for stage III colon cancer. J Natl Cancer Inst 93:850–857

Schrag D, Rifas-Shiman S, Saltz L et al (2002) Adjuvant chemotherapy use for Medicare beneficiaries with stage II colon cancer. J Clin Oncol 20:3999–4005

Schuller J, Cassidy J, Dumont E et al (2000) Preferential activation of capecitabine in tumor following oral administration to colorectal cancer patients. Cancer Chemother Pharmacol 45:291–297

Seow A, Koh WP, Chia KS et al (2004) Trends in cancer incidence in Singapore 1968–2002. Singapore Cancer Registry Report no. 6

Seymour MT, Thompson LC, Wasan HS et al (2011) Chemotherapy options in elderly and frail patients with metastatic colorectal cancer (MRC FOCUS2): an open-label, randomised factorial trial. Lancet 377:1749–1759

Singapore Cancer Registry (2005–2009) Interim Annual Registry Report 2005–2009. National Registry of Diseases Office

Singapore Department of Statistics (2011) Population trends. ISSN 1793 2424

Stein BN, Petrelli NJ, Douglass HO et al (1995) Age and sex are independent predictors of 5-fluorouracil toxicity. Analysis of a large scale phase III trial. Cancer 75:11–17

Sundararajan V, Mitra N, Jacobson JS et al (2002) Survival associated with 5-fluorouracil-based adjuvant chemotherapy among elderly patients with node-positive colon cancer. Ann Intern Med 136:349–357

Tabah-Fisch I, Maindrault-Goebel F, Benavides M et al (2002) Oxaliplatin/5 FU/LV is feasible, safe and active in elderly colorectal cancer (CRC) patients. Proc Am Soc Clin Olcol 21: abstract 556

Tan KY, Konishi F, Suzuki K (2010) The evidence for adjuvant treatment of elderly patients (age ≥ 70) with stage III colon cancer is inconclusive. Surg Today 40:2–3

Tournigand C, Andre T, Bachet J et al (2010) FOLFOX4 as adjuvant therapy in elderly patients (pts) with colon cancer (CC): subgroup analysis of the MOSAIC trial. J Clin Oncol 2(15s): abstract 3522

Tsalic M, Bar-Sela G, Beny A et al (2003) Severe toxicity related to the 5-fluorouracil/leucovorin combination (the Mayo Clinic regimen): a prospective study in colorectal cancer patients. Am J Clin Oncol 26:103–106

Twelves C, Wong A, Nowacki MP et al (2005a) Capecitabine as adjuvant treatment for stage III colon cancer. N Engl J Med 352:2696–2704

Twelves CJ, Butts CA, Cassidy J et al (2005b) Capecitabine/oxaliplatin, a safe and active first-line regimen for older patients with metastatic colorectal cancer: post hoc analysis of a large phase II study. Clin Colorectal Cancer 5:101–107

Twelves C, Scheithauer W, McKendrick J et al (2011) Capecitabine versus 5-fluorouracil/folinic acid as adjuvant therapy for stage III colon cancer: final results from the X-ACT trial with analysis by age and preliminary evidence of a pharmacodynamic marker of efficacy. Ann Oncol. doi:10.1093/annonc/mdr366

Van Cutsem E, Hoff PM, Harper P et al (2004) Oral capecitabine vs intravenous 5-fluorouracil and leucovorin: integrated efficacy data and novel analyses from two large, randomised, phase III trials. Br J Cancer 90:1190–1197

Van Cutsem E, Labianca R, Bodoky G et al (2009) Randomized phase III trial comparing biweekly infusional fluorouracil/leucovorin alone or with irinotecan in the adjuvant treatment of stage III colon cancer: PETACC-3. J Clin Oncol 27:3117–3125

Wieland D, Hirth V (2003) Comprehensive geriatric assessment. Cancer Control 10:454–462

Yancik R (2005) Population aging and cancer: a cross-national concern. Cancer J 11:437–441

Yancik R, Ries LA (2004) Cancer in older persons: an international issue in an aging world. Semin Oncol 31:128–136

Ychou M, Raoul JL, Douillard JY et al (2009) A phase III randomised trial of LV5FU2 + irinotecan versus LV5FU2 alone in adjuvant high-risk colon cancer (FNCLCC Accord02/FFCD9802). Ann Oncol 20:674–680

Yellen SB, Cella DF, Leslie WT (1994) Age and clinical decision making in oncology patients. J Natl Cancer Inst 86:1766–1770

Zalcberg J, Kerr D, Seymour L et al (1998) Haematological and non-haematological toxicity after 5-fluorouracil and leucovorin in patients with advanced colorectal cancer is significantly associated with gender, increasing age and cycle number. Tomudex International Study Group. Eur J Cancer 34:1871–1875

Zuckerman IH, Rapp T, Onukwugha E et al (2009) Effect of age on survival benefit of adjuvant chemotherapy in elderly patients with stage III colon cancer. J Am Geriatr Soc 57:1403–1410

Palliative Care for the Elderly with Colorectal Cancer

16

Woon-Chai Yong, Norhisham bin Main, Song-Chiek Quah,
Laurence Tan, and James Low

Take Home Pearls

- Markers and tools can aid prognostication of palliative care patients with colorectal cancer; progressive loss of performance is an important marker.
- Disease control is multimodal and also includes symptomatic control.
- Symptoms commonly encountered are pain, bowel obstruction, and bleeding.
- Psychosocial and spiritual distress in palliative care patients need to be addressed with empathy.
- Advance care planning is good practice in palliation.

16.1 Introduction

Colorectal carcinoma is a common condition in the developed countries. Cancer was the second leading cause of death in United States in 2010, and among these, colorectal cancer was the second most common cause of mortality (American Cancer Society 2011). In 2011, it is estimated that there were 141,210 new cases of colorectal cancer and 49,380 deaths occurring from the disease in the United States (Siegel et al. 2011).

W.-C. Yong (✉) • N. bin Main • L. Tan • J. Low
Department of Geriatrics, Palliative Medicine, Khoo Teck Puat Hospital,
90 Yishun Central, Singapore 768828, Singapore
e-mail: yong.woon.chai@alexandrahealth.com.sg; main.norhisham@alexandrahealth.com.sg;
tan.laurence.lc@alexandrahealth.com.sg; low.james.yh@alexandrahealth.com.sg

S.-C. Quah
Radiation Oncology, National Cancer Center,
11, Hospital Drive 169610, Singapore
e-mail: daniel.quah.s.c@nccs.com.sg

K.-Y. Tan (ed.), *Colorectal Cancer in the Elderly*,
DOI 10.1007/978-3-642-29883-7_16, © Springer-Verlag Berlin Heidelberg 2013

Over the last 20 years, the treatment outcome of colorectal cancer has improved dramatically. This is in tandem with the development of general medical science. Despite this, there is an increasing need for the care of colorectal cancer patients who are unable to participate in curative treatments. Approximately 20% of patients already have metastatic disease on presentation which would preclude them from curative treatments. On the other hand, up to about 40% of treated patients develop recurrences, and further curative treatments are often deemed unsuitable (Rothenberger 2004). There are also a significant portion frail elderly with technically resectable colorectal tumor who are unfit for curative or aggressive treatment in view of their poor performance status or comorbidities. In such instances, palliative care is most appropriate for these patients.

The term palliative care is derived from the original Latin root word palliare meaning "to cloak." Palliative care aims to improve the quality of life and reduce the suffering of patients and their family. The concept of palliation has been evolving over the last decade. The intent of palliative treatment can be disease control, symptoms control, or both, so long as it achieves the goal of comfort.

Many reports have suggested unmet physical or emotional needs in patient with advanced colorectal cancer. This has led to the advocating of early access to palliative service. SIGN (Scottish Intercollegiate Guidelines Network) guideline currently recommends that prompt referral to palliative services be made in colorectal cancer patients with complicated symptoms control.

16.2 Prognostication

> Declare the past, diagnose the present, foretell the future.
> – Hippocrates

Prognostication means to predict according to present indications or signs. Here, we shall limit the discussion to survival prediction.

Prognostication is important to patients, their family, and the healthcare professionals to decide on goals and extent of treatment. While prognostication will affect choices of treatment, treatment may also change the outcome of the illness. The interaction between them is often beyond any prognostic tools. Communication of the limitations of prognostic tools to the patient and their family is of paramount importance.

16.2.1 Prognostic Markers and Tools

In general, it is more challenging to predict survival in locally advanced colorectal cancer than in metastatic disease. In untreated metastatic colorectal disease, the median survival is 5 months (Scheithauer 1993). Further prognostication in metastatic disease is related to the location and extent of metastasis, as well as the momentum of decline.

Patients who are symptomatic upon diagnosis usually have worse prognosis (Copeland et al. 1968; Beahrs and Sanfelippo 1971). Many symptoms, including obstruction, perforation, anorexia, dysphagia, confusion, dyspnea, xerostomia, and malignant ascites are associated with poor outcome.

Toward the later stages of the disease, the single most important predictive factor of mortality is progressive loss of performance status. Patients with solid tumors typically lose ~70% of their functional ability in the last 3 months of life. One of the commonly used models is Palliative Performance Status (Lau et al. 2006), which comprises of the following five domains:

- Patient's ability to ambulate
- Patient's activity and evidence of disease
- Patient's ability to care for self
- Patient's level of food intake
- Patient's level of consciousness

While there are no clear consensuses as to which predictive scale is the most accurate, our clinical experiences show that the use of Palliative Performance Status in palliative patients is accurate and simple to use.

16.2.2 Communication of Prognosis

As mentioned above, communication of the prognosis is of upmost importance in view of the variances that may be expected when calculating survival predictions. A four-step approach to discussing prognostication was described in End of Life/ Palliative Education Resource Center (EPERC):

- Confirm the readiness to hear prognostic information.
- Present information using a range: days to weeks, weeks to short months, etc.
- Allow silence after provision of information, response to emotion.
- Use prognostic information as a starting point for eliciting end-of-life goals.

16.3   Disease Control

For the elderly with colorectal cancer treated with palliative intent, interventions fall into two broad, and occasionally overlapping, groups – those that hope to control the course of disease, such as palliative chemotherapy, and those that control symptoms.

16.3.1 Palliative Chemotherapy

Advances in the recent decades in chemotherapeutics as well as in targeted therapies have brought about a nearly quadrupling of the median survival of patients with metastatic colorectal cancer. A detailed discussion of systemic therapy for unresectable metastatic colorectal cancer is beyond the scope of this chapter. As such, only a brief summary shall be attempted. The reader is referred to other chapters for discussion of the management of potentially resectable metastatic colorectal cancer (see Chap. 16).

- With only supportive care, patients with metastatic colorectal cancer have a median overall survival (MOS) of about 6 months.
- Fluoropyrimidine monotherapies confer an increase in MOS to the order of 10–12 months (Cochrane Database 2000).

- The oral derivative of fluoropyrimidine, capecitabine (Xeloda, Roche), is as effective as the intravenous version, 5-fluorouracil (5-FU) (Van Cutsem et al. 2004).
- Fluoropyrimidine-based doublet combination chemotherapy regimes result in the addition of further increase in MOS to around 17 months. Such regimes include FOLFOX, using Oxaloplatin, a platinum-based alkylating agent (de Gramont et al. 2000), and FOLFIRI, using irinotecan, a topoisomerase inhibitor (Saltz et al. 2000).
- The strategy of using all three agents – 5-fluorouracil, oxaloplatin, and irinotecan – conferred a MOS of 21 months (Tournigand et al. 2004).
- The addition of targeted agents to doublet chemotherapy also yielded a similar median overall survival, for example:
  - Bevacizumab (Avastin, Genentech/Roche) is a monoclonal antibody against vascular endothelial growth factor ligand. When added to a doublet of 5-FU and irinotecan, it yielded a MOS of 20.3 months (Hurwitz et al. 2004).
  - Cetuximab (Erbitux, Merck) is an epidermal growth factor receptor monoclonal antibody. The CRYSTAL trial showed an increase in MOS to 23.5 months, when cetuximab added to FOLFIRI (van Cutsem et al. 2009).

The efficacy of palliative chemotherapy in fit elderly patients with unresectable metastatic colorectal cancer was obtained mainly from subgroup analyses of studies including those above, which showed that this group of patients achieved similar benefits as their younger counterparts. The reader is referred to the chapter "Adjuvant Chemotherapy for Senior Patients after Resection of Colon Cancer" for a discussion on the toxicities of treatment.

In summary, patients should discuss with their oncologist as to which of the above options is the most appropriate, after evaluation of multiple factors which include the patient's physical condition and their personal preferences and beliefs. In general, fit elderly patients with profiles similar to those enrolled in trials should be treated with combination chemotherapy. In the frail elderly patient, chemotherapy should be avoided. As for those who are neither fit nor frail, individualized treatment, such as monotherapy, should be offered after discussion of the pros and cons.

16.3.2 Palliative Radiotherapy

Radiotherapy is the use of ionizing radiation to treat cancer. The most widely used ionizing radiation currently is X-ray. Radiotherapy can be used to treat locally advanced rectal tumors in elderly patients who decline surgical interventions for personal or medical reasons.

X-ray beams have to traverse normal tissue to reach the tumor, and it is the dose deposited in these normal tissues that result in side effects. The dose-limiting organ for radiotherapy of rectal tumors is the small bowel, which can only tolerate doses up to the order of 45–50 Gy. As such, the dose deliverable to rectal tumor is usually limited to 45 Gy in 25 fractions. Some radiation oncologists prefer to deliver an additional boost of up to 9 Gy in for a total of 54 Gy in 30 fractions, with the opinion that a higher dose may have better local control. Both treatment doses, however, are considered insufficient for tumoricidal effects and thus are aimed for controlling the disease locally.

With the advent of newer technology in radiotherapy, both in terms of imaging as well as newer radiation with better beam profile, it may be possible in the future to deliver higher tumor dose with a lower normal-tissue exposure, which in turn leads to even better local control, with lesser side effects.

16.4   Symptoms and Symptoms Management

Symptoms development in colorectal cancer may be generalized symptoms or specific to the tumor. There are a wide range of possible symptoms which can emerge in the course of the disease. In this section, we shall focus on 3 common symptoms that colorectal cancer patients may experience: pain, intestinal obstruction, and bleeding.

A commonly used validated symptom assessment tool is the Revised Edmonton Symptom Scoring System (ESAS). It is useful in both clinical and research setting (Watanabe et al. 2011).

16.4.1 Pain

> In order to understand the Pain, you have to know the Patient (as a Person) and the Pathology.
> – WC Yong

IASP (International Association for the Study of Pain) defines pain as an unpleasant sensory and emotional experience associated with actual or potential tissue damage, or described in terms of such damage. Cancer pain, especially in the elderly, is common and may be complex in nature. The nature of pain experienced may be nociceptive, neuropathic, or a combination of the above.

Many elderly may under report the severity and prevalence of pain. Therefore, cancer pain assessment is the key to guiding treatment decision. A detailed pain history is essential. There are various pain assessment tools available, which may be unidimensional (e.g., visual analogue scale, numerical rating scale) or multidimensional (e.g., The Brief Pain Inventory, the McGill Pain Questionnaire).

16.4.1.1 Pain Assessment

Pain assessment can be challenging in the presence of cognitive impairment and communication difficulties, which is common among the elderly. Some studies described impaired ability to complete and comprehend self-report pain rating scales among persons with MMSE below 15. Various objective pain assessment tools have been developed for such settings. Most of the tools include observation of nonverbal cues in pain expression, for example, agitation, shouting, and grimacing. Understanding

| Edmonton symptom assessment system: |
| Numerical scale |
| Regional palliative care program |

Please circle the number that describes:

Not pain   0 1 2 3 4 5 6 7 8 9 10 Worst possible pain

Not tired   0 1 2 3 4 5 6 7 8 9 10 Worst possible tiredness

Not nauseated   0 1 2 3 4 5 6 7 8 9 10 Worst possible nausea

Not depressed   0 1 2 3 4 5 6 7 8 9 10 Worst possible depression

Not anxious   0 1 2 3 4 5 6 7 8 9 10 Worst possible anxiety

Not drowsy   0 1 2 3 4 5 6 7 8 9 10 Worst possible drowsiness

Best appetite   0 1 2 3 4 5 6 7 8 9 10 Worst possible appetite

Best feeling of Wellbeing   0 1 2 3 4 5 6 7 8 9 10 Worst possible feeling of wellbeing

No shortness of breath   0 1 2 3 4 5 6 7 8 9 10 Worst possible shortness of breath

Other problem   0 1 2 3 4 5 6 7 8 9 10

Patient's name _____

Date _____ Time _____

Complete by (cheak one)
☐ Patient
☐ Caregiver
☐ Caregiver assisted

Edmonton symptom assessment scale (Reproduced with permission from Edmonton Regional Palliative Care Program)

the baseline characteristics and behavior in a cognitively impaired patient and comparing the changes may be the most important in pain assessment. A number of these tools were developed based on the patient with dementia.

Examples of commonly used pain assessment tools in cognitively impaired patients:

The ABBEY Pain Scale
CNPI (The Checklist of Nonverbal Pain Indicators)
DOLOPLUS-2

PACSLAC (Pain Assessment Checklist for Seniors with Limited Ability to Communicate)
PAINAD (Pain Assessment in Advance Dementia)

16.4.1.2 Pain Management

Pain management can be pharmacological and non-pharmacological in nature. We recommend pharmacological treatment approach based on WHO analgesia ladder. In view of age-related change in organ functions and/or comorbidities in the elderly, choices and dosages of medications have to be tailored according to individual's need and characteristics. Frequent assessment on adequacy of pain control and side effects of medication is imperative. Non-pharmacological methods that may be employed includes heat or cold therapy, music or art therapy, or acupuncture therapy.

16.4.2 Bowel Obstruction

Bowel obstruction occurs when the passage of the intestinal luminal contents is impaired due to a mechanical obstruction or a motility disorder. The obstruction may be partial or complete with an acute or insidious onset. The site of obstruction may be in single or multiple areas. It is reported to occur in 10–28% of advanced gastrointestinal cancer patients.

A consensus committee in 2007 defined the criteria for malignant bowel obstruction. This includes clinical evidence of bowel obstruction with obstruction beyond the ligament of Treitz, on a background of an incurable intra-abdominal primary cancer or a non-intra-abdominal primary cancer with intraperitoneal involvement (Anthony et al. 2007).

16.4.2.1 Pathophysiology of Bowel Obstruction

Bowel obstruction may be mechanical or functional in nature. Mechanical obstruction may arise due to an occlusion of the bowel lumen either extrinsically, intramurally, or intraluminally. The primary tumor itself or tumor deposits on the peritoneum, omentum, or mesentery may cause extrinsic compression of the lumen. Polypoid tumor lesions within the lumen and mural spread of the tumor cause intraluminal and intramural occlusion respectively. A functional obstruction occurs when there is tumor invasion into the neural plexus, or bowel muscle or nerves. It may also result from a paraneoplastic process. In most instances, more than one mechanism may account for the bowel obstruction (Hanks et al. 2011).

16.4.2.2 Making the Diagnosis of Bowel Obstruction

The patient presenting with bowel obstruction may have a history of nausea, vomiting, increasing abdominal distension with or without pain, and a reduced bowel output. There may be a preceding history of previous intestinal obstruction. Clinical examination will reveal the presence of a distended abdomen, and dilated bowel loops may be discernable in thin patients. Palpation may precipitate pain and auscultation may reveal absent or hyperactive bowel sounds.

Plain radiographs of the abdomen will reveal air-fluid levels and can sometimes help determine the level of obstruction. An erect chest X-ray may be required to rule out a perforated bowel resulting from the obstruction (Thomson et al. 2007).

Computed tomogram of the abdomen provides more answers to the cause, severity, site, and complications related to the bowel obstruction. Thus, they are now more commonly ordered for patients presenting with a first episode of bowel obstruction (Suri et al. 1999; Silva et al. 2009).

16.4.2.3 Management of Bowel Obstruction

Bowel obstruction may be managed surgically or medically. The medical management can be further divided into pharmacological and non-pharmacological measures.

Surgical intervention options for bowel obstruction have evolved over the years. The options include percutaneous decompression, endoscopic stenting, diverting stoma creation, and laparoscopic or open resection of affected bowel segments (Tang et al. 1995; Woolfson et al. 1997; Krouse et al. 2002). The decision for surgical intervention should consider factors like performance status, nutritional status, existing comorbidities, intercurrent illness, previous treatment interventions, psychological well-being, social support, extent and grade of the cancer, expected prognosis, and technical feasibility of surgical intervention. Advanced age on its own confers a worse prognosis (Helyer and Easson 2008). If the patient is not a surgical candidate, then aggressive medical management should be instituted (Ripamonti et al. 1993).

The non-pharmacological measure involves the temporary insertion of a nasogastric tube for gastric decompression which is removed when drainage is minimal. This reduces luminal contents of the gut and provides some relief from distension. Long-term placement of a nasogastric tube is strongly discouraged as it is uncomfortable for patients and complications like nasopharyngeal irritation or tube occlusion may occur. Medical management without the use of nasogastric tubes has previously been reported to be successful; hence, nasogastric tubes should be judiciously used (Baines et al. 1985; Ripamonti et al. 2001).

Pharmacological interventions include the use of antisecretory agents, anticholinergics, antihistamines, neuroleptics, and corticosteroids. Some studies have shown the important role of antisecretory agents in the early management of bowel obstruction (Mercadante et al. 1997). Octreotide is a synthetic somatostatin analogue that not only reduces gastrointestinal secretions but also has an antiemetic effect (Ripamonti et al. 2004). However, the cost of the drug may be prohibitive.

There are case reports that the addition of an anticholinergic drug-like scopolamine butylbromide with an antisecretory agent further reduces the secretions and facilitates removal of nasogastric tubes (Mercadante et al. 2004). Anticholinergics may increase mouth dryness and in the elderly can cause confusion and acute urinary retention. The anticholinergics also reduce the colicky abdominal pain associated with bowel obstruction due to its antispasmodic effect on intestinal smooth muscle (Frank 1997).

Vomiting and nausea associated with bowel obstruction are common. Different drugs that target the different pathways and receptors can be used to relieve these symptoms (Ventafridda et al. 1990). Antihistamines like cyclizine and dimenhydrinate are effective in relieving the associated symptoms of nausea and vomiting. They are sometimes used as first-line treatment for vomiting due to bowel obstruction and may be used with other antiemetics. Neuroleptics like haloperidol and chlorpromazine have similarly been shown to be effective. They act on different receptors both centrally and peripherally. Caution should be exercised when combining the use of these drugs with others in the elderly (Frank 1997; Hanks et al. 2011).

Corticosteroids are used to reduce obstruction that may be attributable to edema around the tumor and intestinal wall. Previous studies have reported its effectiveness, and a systematic review showed a trend toward improvement with the use of corticosteroids (Freur et al. 1999).

Prokinetic agents like metoclopramide and domperidone may be considered for use if the obstruction is incomplete. Another pharmacological measure to consider is the use of laxatives either to clear existing fecal impaction or to prevent secondary impaction (Mercadante et al. 1997).

Opioids are known to be effective for pain due to abdominal distension or tumor masses. They should be prescribed to achieve adequate analgesia for pain related to bowel obstruction (Ventafridda et al. 1990). The choice of opioids should take into consideration previous opioid use and existing impairments in liver or renal function.

It is likely that several drugs will be required to achieve symptom control and to attempt reversal of the bowel obstruction. In the elderly, such polypharmacy may result in adverse effects. Thus, drugs should be careful titrated for effect with close monitoring for side effects (Papamichael et al. 2009; Lees and Chan 2011).

In summary, surgical intervention should be considered for suitable patients. Aggressive medical therapy should be given to all patients. Polypharmacy may be unavoidable but adverse events may be reduced with careful dose titration and patient monitoring.

16.4.3 Gastrointestinal Bleeding

Bleeding is a common problem in patients with colorectal tumors. The reader is referred to a review by Pereira and Phan on the management of bleeding in tumors (Pereira and Phan 2004). What follows is a discussion of the interaction between peculiarities unique to the elderly population and selected modes of management detailed in the review article suitable for use in colorectal cancer.

16.4.3.1 Local Therapies
• Packings with or without hemostatic agents
  In colorectal cancer, their use is limited to the rectum, as the more proximal portions of the colon are not accessible without endoscopy.

- Radiotherapy
  The noninvasive nature of radiotherapy makes it a very attractive option for elderly patients. However, the logistics of traveling to and from the radiotherapy center somewhat negates this attractiveness.
  Radiotherapy has been used to arrest bleeding in the rectum and, to a lesser extent, the caecum. A typical dose, in patients with metastatic disease, is 20 Gy in 5 fractions or a single fraction of 8 Gy; either of which would achieve hemostasis in up to 85% of patients. In these sites, patients may be treated with a comfortably full bladder, which displaces most of the relatively more radiosensitive small bowels out of the treatment field.
  Conventional X-ray radiotherapy is not traditionally used on tumors in other parts of the colon, most likely because of the inability to avoid irradiating small bowels. In addition, the intraperitoneal transverse and sigmoid colon are mobile, and thus their position may change quite remarkably during treatment. However, newer radiotherapy techniques may allow better targeting of tumors and, in the future, allow treatment of these portions of the colon.
- Endoscopic techniques
  Local ablation of the tumor is another way of achieving hemostasis.
  This however is limited to patients who can tolerate endoscopic procedures as well as the accompanying sedation.
- Interventional radiology
  Hemostasis can be achieved by using transcutaneous arterial techniques to identify the blood vessel supplying the affected site and then applying a hemostatic agent to that site.
  In the elderly population, patient selection for such procedures need to be very meticulous as their renal function may be impaired and thus making such interventions via fluoroscopy unsuitable.

16.4.3.2 Systemic Therapies

- Correction of coagulopathies
  Blood investigations including full blood count and a coagulation profile may identify abnormalities that may be reversed with replacement blood products.
  Elderly patients may be on antithrombotic prophylaxis such as warfarin and aspirin. Considerations should be made to stop these medications.
- Antifibrinolytic agents
  These include tranexamic acid, a synthetic antifibrinolytic agent that inhibits the conversion of plasminogen into plasmin, which results in a decrease lysis of fibrin clots.
  However, caution is to be exercised if the patient is on antithrombotic prophylaxis, as this may result in fatal blood clots. There should be a detailed discussion between the patient and the attending physician to weigh the risks and benefits of initiating antifibrinolytic agents and continuing antithrombotic prophylaxis.
    Ultimately, prior to initiating any of these managements, it is most important to establish a plan of care consistent with the patient's physical condition and his or her expressed goals.

16.5   Psychological and Spiritual Issues

16.5.1 Depression

Depression is common in patients with advanced cancers. Depressive symptoms can occur in 15–50% while major depression (using the various diagnostic criteria) can occur in 5–20% of such patients (Rosenstein 2011; Tada et al. 2012). Depression occurs as part of the grieving process, especially when a patient faces imminent death. This may have an adverse impact on the patient's quality of life. It may exacerbate the patients suffering, increase the severity of symptoms such as pain, and lead to a desire for hastened death (Breitbart et al. 2000).

There are numerous tools and scales that are used to diagnose and measure depression. In general, the symptoms of depression can be classified broadly into the following categories of the biopsychosocial model of care:

1. Physical symptoms which include loss of weight, loss of appetite, insomnia, fatigue, and generalized weakness
2. Psychological/affective symptoms such as feelings of worthlessness, hopelessness, guilt, being a burden, meaninglessness, and suicidal thoughts
3. Behavioral symptoms (signs) such as psychomotor retardation, tearing, passivity, parasuicide, and perpetual frowning. In advance cancers, the latter two categories should be given more weight when diagnosing depression.

The management of depression in end-of-life care is extremely difficult as the precipitating cause, i.e., the terminal condition itself is invariably irreversible. It requires a multidimensional approach and can be divided into pharmacological and non-pharmacological measures. The non-pharmacological measures should be attempted in the first instance and may have to be supplemented with pharmacological treatment.

The holistic management of depression should include the following:

1. Intensive management of distressing symptoms such as pain and dyspnea
2. Counseling and psychotherapy (e.g., cognitive behavioral therapy, interpersonal therapy) by a psychologist or social worker
3. Engaging the family in the care and support of the patient
4. Social engagement
5. Addressing spiritual and existential pain
6. The use of antidepressants
   The most commonly used antidepressants in terminal illness are the following:
1. Selective serotonin reuptake inhibitors (SSRI), for example, fluoxetine, fluvoxamine, escitalopram, paroxetine, and sertraline
2. Serotonin noradrenaline receptor blockers, for example, mirtazapine
3. Tricyclic antidepressants, for example, nortriptyline and amitriptyline
4. Serotonin noradrenaline reuptake inhibitors (SNRI), for example, venlafaxine
5. The monoamine oxidase inhibitors (MAOI), for example, moclobemide

These antidepressants are selected based on their sedating or activating properties, side effect profile, interaction with other medications, and other ancillary properties. As examples, patients with depression and neuropathic pain could be given a tricyclic antidepressant while those with poor appetite may benefit from mirtazapine. It is important to note though that the above drugs may take between 4 and 6 weeks to act and thus may not be in time for those who have shorter prognoses. Some palliative care physicians and psychiatrists use the psychostimulant, methylphenidate, to overcome this problem. However, it should not be given with tricyclic antidepressants and MAOIs and those with liver impairment, cardiac arrhythmias, and seizures.

Patients with agitation and psychotic symptoms associated with their depression may require neuroleptics at times. The use of electroconvulsive therapy is rare in advanced cancers. However, it may be used as a measure of last resort for those with longer life expectancies and better performance status.

16.5.2 Collusion and Breaking Bad News

Collusion occurs when two parties (the healthcare team and the patient's relatives) make a secret agreement to hide information (the patient's diagnosis or medical condition) from a third party (the patient). This practice is the default position taken in many societies, especially among Asian countries, and goes against some basic ethical principles such as the principle of autonomy, the right to self-determination, truthfulness, and fidelity and the right to medical confidentiality (Low et al. 2009). Collusion also results in suboptimal treatment for the patient who may be deprived of cancer-revealing treatment such as radiotherapy and chemotherapy. Moreover, the patient's lack of knowledge will hinder the patient from making appropriate plans for the limited time he has left in this world and after death. He may be deprived of the opportunity to make a will and advance care planning (see below).

There are many reasons why many well-intentioned families would want collusion. They are being protective toward the patient and believe that knowing the severity of the disease and diagnoses will lead to depression, suicide, a hastened death, hopelessness, and pain.

The act of collusion, however, causes significant burden to the patient, the family, and the attending clinicians. It leads to a breakdown of trust and causes communication barriers between the patient, clinician, and family, who may have to lie and deceive to hide the diagnosis at a time when truth and honesty are most needed.

Collusion should be addressed in most instances and resolved quickly. It should be part and parcel of any good palliative care assessment and management. There are only rare occasions, when revealing the truth may do more harm than good to the patient. And there are instances when revealing the truth would be futile, for example, in severe cognitive impairment.

The suggested approach to resolving collusion is as follows:
1. Understand from the family why they are choosing collusion. Show empathy.
2. Go through with the family the problems and burdens of hiding the diagnosis from the patient.

3. Tell the family that the patient has the right to know and may indeed ask for the truth. If the patient had already expressed the wish to know the diagnosis, this should be made known to the family.
4. Sometimes, it may help to ask the patient if he was "the type who liked to take charge and know everything about himself."
5. Inform the family that there is a technique of breaking bad news (see below). Offer to teach the family if they wish to break the news to the patient themselves.
6. Explain to the family some of the possible initial reactions to the truth, which will almost certainly be not good, but with time and with the family's support, patients will be able to cope and come to terms with the diagnosis. The five stages of grief may apply here.
7. Always reassure the family that the healthcare team will support them as well as the patient right to the end.

Breaking bad news is a skill that is very important in the area of oncology and palliative care. It is an important undertaking that has grave consequences for the patient. It should be undertaken with utmost care and compassion. The act of revealing the diagnosis of an underlying cancer is akin to passing a "death sentence" to a patient; it changes the life and world of the patient and how he views it forever.

A brief summary of some steps to take when breaking bad news is as follows:

1. All the rules for good communication applies, that is, the correct setting, privacy, and communication at eye level.
2. Pace the disclosure slowly and at the patient's pace. The skilled clinician should be able to discern how much and how far to go in the revelation.
3. A warning shot may be required. It sets the scene and pace.
4. Avoid euphemisms.
5. Listen to the patient with your ears and eyes. Give him your "presence."
6. Show empathy and compassion.
7. Almost promise the patient that you would be there for him.
8. At all cost, do not destroy hope. Hope may be redirected to something apart from a cure. It could be to complete tasks, for a painless death, and other foreseeable targets.

16.5.3 Spirituality

This is the dimension of the human that deals with existential issues and takes on a larger significance in those at the end of life. It has to do with the meaning and value one ascribes to events, persons, life, death, illness, etc. It is connectedness to something beyond oneself. It seeks answers and is the quest for ultimate ends. Spirituality is the concern of every human being regardless of whether he or she has a religion. Religiosity on the other hand is a means in which people find answers to some of the existential questions of life.

For patients with advanced cancers, the questions are framed against the past, present, and the future. In the past, patients will ask questions such as the following: "What did I do to deserve this?" "Is this retribution from God?" "If only I had gone for that screening at the clinic" Questions centered on the present will include the following: "Why me?" "Why now?" "Why is there so much pain and suffering?" "What is the meaning of this illness?" "I wish I was dead!" While toward the future, the patient will worry about what type of death he would experience, what would become of his loved ones, and what would there be beyond this life. Such concerns are manifested in questions such as the following: "Is there life after death?" "What would it feel like to move from a state of existence to nonexistence or extinction?" (Tan 2007). Fear of the unknown is what makes dying frightening to the human person.

Spiritual pain can have a negative impact on the well-being and quality of life of the patient.

Clinicians have much difficulty managing spiritual issues in dying cancer patients. We feel ill-equipped to manage such complex and delicate matters. However, the following approach could be adopted:

1. Show empathy even if we are unable to help much. Be there for the patient.
2. Do not impose one's values or be judgmental toward the patient.
3. Again, maintenance of hope is extremely essential.
4. Understand the importance of religion in the patients approach to life.
5. Offer to refer the patient to a pastoral care worker, chaplain, or social worker.
6. Offer to refer the patient to his or her religious clergy.
7. Assist the patient in making advance care plans which is aligned partly to good spiritual care (see below).

16.6 Advance Care Planning

Advance care planning (ACP) refers to a process whereby a patient expresses his views, values, wishes, preferences, and goals toward treatment and care as he approaches the end of life. This process also requires the patient to appoint a surrogate decision maker or to make a Lasting Power of Attorney (LPA) in case he loses the capacity to make decisions for himself.

In patients with advanced cancers, the need to make advance care planning becomes urgent. ACP can be carried out in many ways, via, for example, an advance medical directive or living will, a values history, a personal note, etc. A good system incorporates elements of all the above means. Making an ACP will help the family and healthcare team make decisions that are in line with the wishes and goals of the patient and in accordance with his religious and cultural beliefs even at the time when the patient has lost his ability to make and communicate decisions about his care and management. Most ACP systems for terminally ill patients will require the following process (Briggs and Hammes 2011):

1. The patient should be aware of the diagnosis and prognosis.
2. He should also be aware of all the treatment options available, the risk and benefit involved, and the possible outcomes of the various interventions.

3. The patient should be given the opportunity to reflect and think over the information that is provided. He may wish to discuss with his loved one. At this stage, a form or booklet can be given to guide him in his thinking.
4. A willing surrogate decision maker who knows the patient well should be identified and appointed.
5. It is preferable that the patient expresses his wishes and documents it.
6. This document should then be made available to the patient, his surrogate decision maker, and the healthcare teams that are managing or are expected to manage him in future.
7. His wishes should also be translated into a physician order.

Conclusion

Palliative care is the total care of patient with life-limiting disease and their families. Multidisciplinary care involvement may be crucial as it involves integration of physical, psychosocial, and spiritual aspect. It is about healing. Often, it is about supporting the patient and family going through the final journey, which leads to closure. We hope that it can be a dignified process. While medical measures may fail, we as professional healthcare providers will do well to remember that our presence and our reassuring words can be the most soothing medicine.

You matter because you are you. You matter to the last moment of your life, and we will do all we can not only to help you die peacefully, but to live until you die
– Saunders C.

References

American Cancer Society (2011) Cancer facts and figures 2011. American Cancer Society, Atlanta. Retrieved December 19, 2011

Anthony T et al (2007) Report of the clinical protocol committee: development of randomized trials for malignant bowel obstruction. J Pain Symptom Manage 34:S49–S59

Baines M et al (1985) Medical management of intestinal obstruction in patients with advanced malignant disease. Lancet 326:990–993

Beahrs OH, Sanfelippo PM (1971) Factors in prognosis of colon and rectal cancer. Cancer 28:213

Breitbart W, Rosenfeld B, Pessin H et al (2000) Depression, hopelessness, and desire for hastened death in terminally ill patients with cancer. JAMA 284(22):2907–2911

Briggs L, Hammes B (2011) Respecting choices – an advance care planning system that works. Gundersen-Lutheran Medical Foundation. http://respectingchoices.org/. Accessed 29 Jan 2012

Cochrane Database Syst Rev (2000) Palliative chemotherapy for advanced or metastatic colorectal cancer: colorectal meta-analysis collaboration. CD001545

Copeland EM, Miller LD, Jones RS (1968) Prognostic factors in carcinoma of the colon and rectum. Am J Surg 116:875

de Gramont A, Figer A, Seymour M et al (2000) Leucovorin and fluorouracil with or without oxaliplatin as first-line treatment in advanced colorectal cancer. J Clin Oncol 18:2938–2947

Frank C (1997) Medical management of intestinal obstruction in terminal care. Can Fam Physician 43:259–265

Freur DJ et al (1999) Systematic review and meta-analysis of corticosteroids for the resolution of malignant bowel obstruction in advanced gynaecological and gastrointestinal cancers. Ann Oncol 10:1035–1041

Hanks G et al (2011) Oxford textbook of palliative medicine, 4th edn. Oxford University Press, Oxford/New York

Helyer L, Easson AM (2008) Surgical approaches to malignant bowel obstruction. J Support Oncol 5:105–113

Hurwitz H, Fehrenbacher L, Novotny W et al (2004) Bevacizumab plus irinotecan, fluorouracil, and leucovorin for metastatic colorectal cancer. N Engl J Med 350:2335–2342

Krouse RS et al (2002) When the sun can set on an unoperated bowel obstruction: management of malignant bowel obstruction. J Am Coll Surg 195:117–128

Lau F, Downing GM, Lesperance M et al (2006) Use of palliative performance scale in end-of-life prognostication. J Palliat Med 9:1066–1075

Lees J, Chan A (2011) Polypharmacy in elderly patients with cancer: clinical implications and management. Lancet Oncol 12:1249–1257

Low JA, Kiow SL, Main N et al (2009) Reducing collusion between family members and clinicians of patients referred to the palliative care team. Perm J 13(4):11–15

Mercadante S et al (1997) Octreotide may prevent definitive intestinal obstruction. J Pain Symptom Manage 13:352–355

Mercadante S et al (2004) Aggressive pharmacological treatment for reversing malignant bowel obstruction. J Pain Symptom Manage 28:412–416

Papamichael D et al (2009) Treatment of the elderly colorectal cancer patient: SIOG expert recommendations. Ann Oncol 20:5–16

Pereira J, Phan T (2004) Management of bleeding in patients with advanced cancer. Oncologist 9:561–570

Ripamonti C et al (1993) Management of bowel obstruction in advanced and terminal cancer patients. Ann Oncol 4:15–21

Ripamonti C et al (2001) Clinical practice recommendations for the management of bowel obstruction in patients with end stage cancer. Support Care Cancer 9:223–233

Ripamonti C et al (2004) Role of octreotide, scopolamine butylbromide and hydration in symptom control of patients with inoperable bowel obstruction and nasogastric tubes: a prospective randomized trial. J Pain Symptom Manage 19:23–34

Rosenstein DL (2011) Depression and end-of-life care for patients with cancer, dialogues. Clin Neurosci 13(1):101–108

Rothenberger DA (2004) Palliative therapy of rectal cancer. Overview: epidemiology, indications, goals, extent, and nature of work-up. J Gastrointest Surg 8:259–261

Saltz LB, Cox JV, Blanke C et al (2000) Irinotecan plus fluorouracil and leucovorin for metastatic colorectal cancer. N Engl J Med 343:905–914

Scheithawer et al (1993) Randomised comparison ot combination plus supportive core with supportive care alone in patients with metastatic colorectal cancer. BMJ 306:752

Siegel R, Ward E, Brawley O et al (2011) Cancer statistics, 2011: the impact of eliminating socioeconomic and racial disparities on premature cancer deaths. CA Cancer J Clin 61:212

Silva AC et al (2009) Small bowel obstruction: what to look for. Radiographics 29:423–439

Suri S et al (1999) Comparative evaluation of plain films, ultrasound and CT in the diagnosis of intestinal obstruction. Acta Radiol 40:422–428

Tada Y, Matsubara M, Kawada S et al (2012) Psychiatric disorders in cancer patients at a University Hospital in Japan: descriptive analysis of 765 psychiatric referrals. Jpn J Clin Oncol 42(3):183–188

Tan YS (2007) Understanding and addressing spiritual distress. S'pore Fam Phys 33(3):69–74

Tang E et al (1995) Bowel obstruction in cancer patients. Arch Surg 130:832–837

Thomson WM et al (2007) Accuracy of abdominal radiography in acute small bowel obstruction: does reviewer experience matter? Am J Roentgenol 188:W233–W238

Tournigand C, Andre T, Achille E et al (2004) FOLFIRI followed by FOLFOX6 or the reverse sequence in advanced colorectal cancer: a randomized GERCOR study. J Clin Oncol 22:229–237

Van Cutsem E, Hoff P, Harper P et al (2004) Oral capecitabine versus intravenous 5-fluorouracil and leucovorin: integrated efficacy data and novel analyses from two large, randomised, phase III trials. Br J Cancer 90:1190–1197

Van Cutsem E, Köhne CH, Hitre E et al (2009) Cetuximab and chemotherapy as initial treatment for metastatic colorectal cancer. N Engl J Med 360(14):1408–1417

Ventafridda V et al (1990) The management of inoperable gastrointestinal obstruction in terminal cancer patients. Tumori 76:389–393

Watanabe SM, Nekolaichuk C, Beaumont C et al (2011) A multi-centre comparison of two numerical versions of the Edmonton Symptom Assessment System in palliative care patients. J Pain Symptom Manage 41:456–468

Woolfson RG et al (1997) Management of bowel obstruction in patients with abdominal cancer. Arch Surg 132:1093–1097

Index

K.-Y. Tan (ed.), *Colorectal Cancer in the Elderly*,
DOI 10.1007/978-3-642-29883-7, © Springer-Verlag Berlin Heidelberg 2013